Praise for CAL OREY
Classic Health Book

The Healing Powers of Superfoods
"Ancient healing wisdom meets modern-day foods in this super book."
—Ann Louise Gittleman, Ph.D., C.N.S.,
author of *The Fat Flush Plan*

"In *The Healing Powers of Superfoods*, we're thankfully
rediscovering these amazingly healthy foods again today."
—Will Clower, Ph.D., CEO, Mediterranean Wellness

The Healing Powers of Tea
"Confirmed enthusiasts of the drink will most appreciate Orey's
well-constructed and comprehensive guide; foodies and those
with an interest in alternative-health therapies will also want
to thumb through it."
—*Publishers Weekly*

"Tea is an ancient elixir that is making quite a therapeutic
comeback. I know this book will be your cup of tea!"
—Ann Louise Gittleman, Ph.D., C.N.S.,
author of *The Fat Flush Plan*

"*The Healing Powers of Tea*, like the drink itself, is a
nourishing comfort."
—Will Clower, Ph.D., CEO, Mediterranean Wellness

The Healing Powers of Vinegar
"A practical, health-oriented book that everyone who wants to stay
healthy and live longer should read."
—Patricia Bragg, N.D., Ph.D., author of *Apple Cider Vinegar*

"Deserves to be included in everybody's kitchen and medicine chest."
—Ann Louise Gittleman, Ph.D., C.N.S.,
author of *The Fat Flush Plan*

"Wonderfully useful for everyone interested in health."
—Elson M. Haas, M.D., author of *Staying Healthy with Nutrition, 21st Century Edition*

The Healing Powers of Olive Oil
"One of the most healing foods on the planet. A fascinating read; olive oil is not only delicious, it is good medicine!"
—Ann Louise Gittleman, Ph.D., C.N.S.,
author of *The Fat Flush Plan*

"Orey gives kudos to olive oil, and people of all ages will benefit from her words of wisdom."
—Will Clower, Ph.D., CEO, Mediterranean Wellness

"Olive oil has been known for centuries to have healing powers and now we know why. It is rich in monounsaturated fats similar to avocado and macadamia nut oils. The information in this book will help you to understand the healing powers of oils."
—Fred Pescatore, M.D., M.P.H., author of *The Hamptons Diet*

The Healing Powers of Coffee
"A cup or two of joe every day is a good way to boost mood, energy, and overall health."
—Julian Whitaker, M.D., founder,
Whitaker Wellness Institute

"For heart, mind, and body, Cal Orey shows us why coffee is the most comforting health food on the planet."
—Dr. Will Clower, Ph.D., CEO, Mediterranean Wellness

"A fascinating read about a natural remedy that is a rich source of antioxidants."
—Ray Sahelian, M.D., author of *Mind Boosters*

"Not everyone can be a beekeeper, but Cal Orey shares the secrets that honeybees and their keepers have always known. Honey is good for body and soul."
—Kim Flottum, editor of *Bee Culture* magazine and author of several honeybee books

The Healing Powers of Chocolate
"The right kind, the right amount of chocolate may just save your life."
—Ann Louise Gittleman, Ph.D., C.N.S., author of *The Fat Flush Plan*

"Chocolate is a taste of divine ecstasy on Earth. It is our sensual communion. Orey's journalistic style and efforts share this insight with readers around the world."
—Jim Walsh, founder, Intentional Chocolate

Books by CAL OREY

The Healing Powers of Tea

The Healing Powers of Coffee

The Healing Powers of Honey

The Healing Powers of Chocolate

The Healing Powers of Olive Oil

The Healing Powers of Vinegar

Doctors' Orders

202 Pets' Peeves

Published by Kensington Publishing Corp.

The
Healing Powers of
Superfoods

A Complete Guide to Nature's Favorite Functional Foods

CAL OREY

CITADEL PRESS
Kensington Publishing Corp,
www.kensingtonbooks.com

CITADEL PRESS BOOKS are published by

Kensington Publishing Corp.
119 West 40th Street
New York, NY 10018

Copyright © 2019 Cal Orey

Permission to reproduce The Mediterranean Diet Pyramid and Common Foods and Flavors of the Mediterranean Diet Pyramid 2009, granted by Oldways Preservation & Trust, www.oldwayspt.org

All Kensington titles, imprints, and distributed lines are available at special quantity discounts for bulk purchases for sales promotions, premiums, fund-raising, educational, or institutional use. Special book excerpts or customized printings can also be created to fit specific needs. For details, write or phone the office of the Kensington sales manager: Kensington Publishing Corp., 119 West 40th Street, New York, NY 10018, attn: Sales Department; phone 1-800-221-2647.

CITADEL PRESS and the Citadel logo are Reg. U.S. Pat. & TM Off.

ISBN-13: 978-0-8065-3898-3
ISBN-10: 0-8065-3898-8

First trade paperback printing: January 2019

10 9 8 7 6 5 4 3

Printed in the United States of America

Library of Congress CIP data is available.

Electronic edition: January 2019

ISBN-13: 978-0-8065-3899-0
ISBN-10: 0-8065-3899-6

A special dedication to three comforting, strong, and steady males in my daily life.
Love, light, and blessings to my younger sibling, Bruce, cat, Zen, and dog, Skyler.
This trio provides balance and energy to my mind and spirit—much like the remarkable healing powers of superfoods.

CONTENTS

Foreword

Change can be disconcerting. Like broken sleep and sudden starts, it definitely gets your attention—for a while, anyway, until you regain your bearings and return to the reality you can count on.

Our food is much the same. It can be startling how the regular parade of faddish dietary schemes seem to change what you're supposed to be eating each year. One year you're throwing out fats, and the next you're throwing out carbs. Egg were awful, now they're fine; margarine would save your life, now it contributes to heart valve problems; and coffee was a carcinogen, and now it fights cancer.

It's like there's some giant *The Price Is Right* "wheel of nutrition" that gets spun and *tick tick ticks* along until it lands on the new gluten or dairy or peanut butter fascination. The list is as exhaustive as it is exhausting.

And like a bad dream, each new food fad alerts your attention until someone takes another spin of the wheel next January and everyone hyperventilates about the next "miraculous" food fetish.

TRADITIONAL SUPERFOODS—THEN AND NOW

By contrast, I reviewed the list of superfoods Cal covers in this work, and felt instantly relieved. It cuts through the spin cycle of annual food fads. I was reminded of growing up in a time when no one was afraid of an egg for breakfast, an apple as a snack, sliced tomatoes for dinner, or maybe watermelon for dessert.

Those family foods live for me like a bright warming memory. And as she points out here in *The Healing Powers of Superfoods*, we're thankfully rediscovering these amazingly healthy foods again today. I say *rediscovering* because we've actually known about them all along. They're not another new fad randomly assigned by the spinning wheel, but a long-established concept of what constitutes our rich heritage of health.

When I lived in France, perhaps the most refreshing aspect of their healthy culture was how much people adhered to their own heritage of health. They were just not distracted by the dietary baubles that distract our attention. They stuck to the knowledge that comes from their history, tradition, and culture, and were rewarded with exceptional health for it.

I remember when people first started noticing the Mediterranean diet, and I wondered out loud what the secret was. Maybe it was the olive oil, maybe the tomatoes or cheeses or whatever. But the irony is that while we were looking for one more magic food to promote for the next year, they were just eating as they always have and, hopefully, always will.

What are they eating? Just scroll down the list of superfoods in the volume you are holding and you'll see: apples, nuts, yogurt, berries, greens, tomatoes, lemons, pasta, and wine.

THE HEALTHIEST FOODS ON EARTH

The foods of the Mediterranean diet are as intuitively correct as the memory of something we just realized we'd forgotten. And these superfoods remain the healthiest foods on Earth, without the need for reinvention, repackaging, or a marketing campaign to sell them as the latest and greatest miracle food.

Fortunately for us, the ancient wisdom of this region is becoming the modern awareness of our own culture. The principles that drove its success for centuries are the same ones that can improve ours today.

Once you introduce these delicious foods back into your life, the Earth may spin and new fads and fake foods will certainly be invented to distract our nutritional attention, but you will know to stick with what is right and true and good. Instead of chasing that endless tail, you'll just eat these real foods and be rewarded with optimal health for it.

So, if you want to eat like the healthiest people on Earth, remember what we have recently forgotten and don't allow yourself to get distracted. Just include these basic superfoods and be in control. Make this practice not just what you decide to do today, but who you become for good.

Then, when the next stupendous, amazing, colossal, revolutionary, astonishing, groundbreaking, wonderful *blah blah blah* comes at you with its marketing campaign, you can return to the superfoods that have always brought optimal health, and always will.

In these chapters, reacquaint yourself with this wisdom. Through these pages, learn what the superfoods are, why they are so good for you, and how to use them in your own home.

Blessings and love to you and your family.

—Will Clower, Ph.D.
CEO, Mediterranean Wellness
Author of *The Fat Fallacy* and
The French Don't Diet Plan

Introduction

So, why did I choose to write a book on superfoods, anyhow? Let me explain how this *Healing Powers* book number seven came to fruition—and take you to the land of superfoods. During a number of springtimes, a season of renewal for Mother Nature, I sent a perennial email pitching the topic of nuts, seeds, and berries to my book editor. While I don't solely eat a Stone Age diet, I do follow a plant-based regime and often munch on "rabbit food" (raw vegetables and fruits that most people claim to be boring grub) after a bakefest or change of seasons and while traveling. These foods taste fresh and clean and detoxify the body and mind, versus scarfing down processed junk food with ingredients a scientist can't pronounce.

Perhaps berries, nuts, and seeds make up a bare-to-the-bones cave-man diet and eating them (especially on a daily basis) is too narrow of a feat for most of us—including me. I love a cup of creamy yogurt, a bowl of hot clam chowder paired with a slice of warm artisanal whole-grain bread, a slice of gourmet pizza, or a stack of blueberry pancakes drizzled with sweet maple syrup. So, my proposed cavewoman-style *Healing Powers* book was put on the back burner, year after year, as I continued to savor juicy strawberries, almonds, sunflower seeds, and pasta with tomatoes and Parmesan cheese.

Then, one day at the local supermarket checkout stand, I scruti-nized the no-nonsense, lean, and healthy-looking middle-aged woman ahead of me in line. Her basket of food items looked like my stuff—nutrient dense organic produce, dairy, and eggs. While waiting in a super long cat's tail type line, I spoke. "Excuse me, ma'am." My eyes met hers. "I'm an author and . . . well, I am wondering. Would you read a book on nuts and berries?" A pregnant pause later, the woman reread her grocery list, looked up at me, removed her glasses, and answered, "I like to read recipes for smoothies. I want real food—fast." I listened. Munching on a handful of nuts, I digested her words. I got it. The health-conscious shopper had a life and a family, and whipping up a superfood blender drink is a quick, efficient way to eat—without frills and whistles.

After email exchanges with my editor about my early-man premise for a book, it was clear. It was time for me to time travel outside of the Paleo days. Enter superfoods. Functional foods such as plant-based ones *and* other classic favorite stuff, like water and yogurt, were put on the editorial table. At last, I landed the tweaked project: This book was written due to finding the right timing and combining a balanced list of superfoods in the heart-healthy Mediterranean diet (the underlying premise in the *Healing Powers* series)—a consistently top-ranked diet for good health.

Born and raised on the West Coast of America, I grew up in a mecca of orchards and surrounded by farms—a place plentiful with functional foods from nature. Once I was given a thumbs-up on book number seven in the *Healing Powers* collection, I was excited because I was given the green light to enter Superfoodsland (a place you go to savor clean food from Mother Nature). I am not an exotic food enthusiast (goji berries and hempseed are not in my kitchen or in this book), so being a "granola girl," I feel entering the world of healing foods from a variety of food groups is a good thing. I eagerly accepted the project and opened my mind to including a balance of timeless and tasty superfoods, comfort food with a cause. As a boomer who lived through the health foodies' era of granola and tofu in the seventies and now face a new century of popular superfoods, it is like I got a gift to be able to share the best of both worlds.

No, I am not a doctor or dietitian, but I am a healthy old-timer health author–journalist who dishes about healing foods to nourish the body, mind, and spirit. Like vinegar, olive oil, chocolate, honey, coffee, and tea—six of my favorite superfoods picks. (I've already written books about all of them, and my vinegar book sold more than a quarter million copies around the globe.) This time around, I began my adventure, once again, in the Golden State—a hub of fruits, vegetables, and nuts, real food you can find at the local supermarket, health food store, farmers' market, and roadside fruit and vegetable stands.

So, as a seasoned baby boomer, a.k.a. a tree hugger, I bring to the table traditional superfoods of yesteryear (for my peers and elders) with a fresh twenty-first-century semiexotic twist (specially tailored for the younger generations). It feels like I've morphed into a sci-fi time traveler in the land of superfoods. I'll show you exactly how and why Superfoodsland is the place to be. Go ahead: Fix a cheese plate (complete with local artisanal cheeses, crackers, bread, and apple slices) or grab a bottle of fruit-infused water. Sit down, cozy up, and take time out to discover the exciting land of superfoods.

Acknowledgments

Thanks go to the superfood companies, big and small, farmers, and progressive-thinking health researchers in the United States and around the world who helped me understand how vital nutrient-dense foods are to our health and well-being.

Not to forget the open-minded medical doctors and nutritionists who understand some foods do deserve the label "superfoods"—especially when there is proof that it goes beyond a label for marketing purpose. When scientific studies and anecdotal evidence from ancient times to the present day show food is nature's medicine, it's time to embrace superfoods for what they are—super!

A heartfelt thanks goes to the Kensington Books team, who are behind me from the beginning to end of each *Healing Powers* book. I am grateful to pen the series, all because of a book on vinegar that finally found its sea legs. I never imagined it would lead to a second book on olive oil—a nice pair—and then to chocolate, and on to a series. And I continue to create the book collection.

The Healing Powers of Superfoods is a gift to a health-nut author from California (a super agricultural state). To be given a ticket to write a book on nutrient-dense food from trees, plants, and the sea is exciting. For more than three decades, I've been writing about health and wellness. Big thanks and hugs to followers of the series and readers of this book who are interested in nature's favorite foods.

Author's Note

This book is intended as a reference tool only. It does not give medical advice. Be sure to consult your doctor or the appropriate health-care professional before starting any new diet or exercise program.

Real recipes, tried and true: The superfood recipes in this book have been tested by me, my family and friends, and/or veteran chefs, bakers, and superfood commercial companies and organizations, big and small. Changing ingredients or using different brands of superfoods or kitchen methods may alter the taste, texture, and presentation of a dish. Plus, culinary palates vary. So use your own judgment and follow your instincts and personal tastes when you create a superfood-infused dish or any superfood recipe.

In the superfoods sections on natural home cures and recipes, a variety of nature's multipurpose favorite foods are often paired. Take precautions regarding personal food allergies, which vary a lot (e.g., allergies to citrus, dairy, eggs, nuts, shellfish, tomatoes, and wheat). Millions of people do have at least one food allergy to one specific food. (As a kid, I had an unpleasant experience with kidney beans. So, I stay clear of all legumes but favor other protein-rich superfoods in my diet.)

Meanwhile, do heed warnings on food item nutrition labels, and when dining out ask your server about the contents of dishes that may contain specific culprits (such as nut oils if you're allergic to nuts). Also, think outside of the food container: Consider a custom-tailored substitute superfood (e.g., noncitrus superfruits, gluten-free foods) so you can use a remedy or recipe without consequences.

In the home cures and recipes, honey, another superfood may be used. WARNING: To avoid infant botulism, do not feed honey to a baby who is younger than one year. Also, do not overuse a superfood to achieve better results.

And note, less is more when eating dairy, shellfish, and sweets. (Moderation and portion control are key because of cholesterol, sodium, sugar, and calories.) All of these favorite superfoods in this book do have nutritional virtues and healing powers backed by scientific evidence, especially when paired with other superfoods and when used in a well-balanced diet. Most important, no one superfood is a cure-all; for instance, eating more seaweed will not provide better or quicker results, but you may get an overdose of iodine.

PART 1

SUPERFOODS

The Power of Superfoods

Let food be thy medicine and medicine be thy food.
—HIPPOCRATES

In my imagination, every weekend morning in our farmhouse in the middle of Central California, surrounded by orchards and groves, I'd sit at a rustic wooden kitchen table. My mother scooped a spoonful of hot oatmeal into my bowl and topped it with fresh raspberries, paired with a side of scrambled eggs and diced tomatoes off the vine. As we ate, she'd dished out daily chores: picking apples and making batches of berry jam for the autumn harvest. Reaping the rewards of nature's finest food was normal to me, a kid at a farmhouse. I often gazed out the kitchen window to hear and see neighbors' roosters and cows roaming on dairy farms. Those were typical days, sort of.

I can almost remember when my leisure-loving grandmother, who traveled the world, visited. During the warm Indian summer night we sat on the porch swing. Nibbling on homemade almond butter cookies and drinking cold lemonade under the harvest moon, she read to me my favorite book, *The Adventures of Tom Sawyer*, beginning with Aunt Polly searching for Tom, discovering the boy had been sneaking jam. This rural paradise slice of life takes me back in time, back to nature, but it's an exaggerated tale.

Truth be told, my real life was a bit of a bore. I could see the Los

Gatos foothills from our sofa next to the living room window—a safe place I'd go and imagine the world I had not experienced. I *was* raised in an agricultural hub, full of plum and apricot orchards, a place where the scent of fruit filled the air when I took walks to the mall with my friends. But there were no eggs to fetch; I just saw that on *The Real McCoys*, a TV show about a family who came out West to become farmers.

But the truth is, I *really* did eat and enjoy superfoods in my youth. I was homegrown in San Jose, California, a place once dubbed "the Valley of Heart's Delight," and I still have images of its natural, whole foods. We'd pick fresh fruits and vegetables from neighbors' yards and nearby orchards, and both lettuce and strawberry fields were thirty miles away from our home. But I was not raised as a farmer's daughter, nor did I raise chickens or collect eggs at the crack of dawn.

Now, as a Golden State–grown health-nut foodie, I can look back at my life growing up, decade by decade, and understand how superfoods played a big role in my real world. I got a feel for farm-to-table meals and the trend of health food store superfoods (avoiding fast food and frozen boxed dinners) with their healing powers throughout my wonder years of growing up in the suburbs.

A Time for Superfoods

Today, after more than a half century of living, I sit here writing in a rustic mountain cabin amid pine trees (minus a dozen due to gentrification). True, I'm not on farmland, but I feel a healthy vibe, surrounded by nature that keeps on giving both beauty and nourishment as I write *The Healing Powers of Superfoods*.

For countless people—and perhaps for you, too—the healing powers of superfoods are no secret. Like me, people use superfoods not only as home cures but also as a weight-loss, heart-healthy, and anti-aging prescription, where they give a health boost by teaming up with herbs and spices.

If you haven't heard by now, listen up. Your health—mind, body, and spirit—may depend on it. Chances are, you, like me, already have superfoods in your kitchen fridge, cupboards, and on the countertops. I'm talking about whole foods—good, clean, edible fare—not processed junk with ingredients you can't pronounce or define.

There is a lot to discover about superfoods that is super and that you need to know about.

The Super Term for Superfood

Superfood: A food that is considered to be very good for your health and that may even help some medical conditions.—*The Macmillan Dictionary*

Medical doctors and even superfood researchers continue to make new findings about superfoods. It's not just about acai and noni. In mainstream America and around the globe, people are discovering just what folk herbalists have been saying throughout history, that nature's finest foods have remarkable healing powers.

Superfood Smoothies author Julie Morris points out that superfood "essentials" in smoothies are chock-full of vitamins and minerals, providing more benefits than other foods and earning their tag "nutritional superheroes."[1]

David Wolfe, author of *Superfoods: The Food of Medicine of the Future* and a raw food guru, also notes, like other clean-food advocates, that superfoods have a baker's dozen of super "unique properties," including being sources of antiaging and immune-boosting antioxidants.[2] These are super substances, such as vitamins, that can prevent chemical reactions that may cause cell damage.

Not to forget *SuperFoods Rx: Fourteen Foods that Will Change Your Life* coauthor Steven G. Pratt, M.D., one of the pioneers who has revolutionized superfoods by educating mainstream Americans in the twentieth century. He explains that the right foods can help you "feel better, have more energy, look better" and halt changes in your body that may lead to disease.[3]

The verdict is in, and it has been evident since the ancient caveman and hunter-gatherer days. Eating a whole foods, natural, plant-based diet is the path to good health and well-being. The best superfoods can and do vary, but despite controversy between the food of the week in the media and scientific nutritional studies backing them, superfoods are functional foods—*not* a gimmick to sell products or a brand despite what some medical doctors believe. Yes, superfoods are real food with super nutrients that provide super healing powers.

MEET THE FAVORITE SUPERFOODS

Today, we know more about the natural goodness behind super-foods—must-have foods to include in your diet. Superfoods—including eggs and Greek yogurt—are considered super medicine that can help your body and mind keep a healthy balance. And this eating-style trend is not a fad, because superfoods can and do help you feel and look better, as well as add super quality years to your life.

Medical researchers believe some antioxidants that act like pharmaceuticals (which are substances that have been manufactured for use as medical drugs while currently being researched for their potential to treat diseases and stall aging) are in superfoods. What's more, superfoods may be super for you and stave off health ailments and diseases. In fact, superfoods have been called "functional foods." And it's no surprise some superfoods are considered super because they are connected with resisting the development of cancer, diabetes, heart disease, and much more.

Ever hear the adage "You are what you eat?" Truth is, you aren't that hot dog and the onion rings you ate at that fast-food drive-thru, but rather what you digest day after day. I learned decades ago that if you eat mid-twentieth-century-style three square meals daily, you still may not be getting enough vitamins and minerals—especially if your dishes are full of processed food that is high in sugar, sodium, and saturated fat. And food researchers will tell you their take on how antioxidant-rich superfoods are superior.

FIVE QUESTIONS FOR JOE VINSON, PH.D.— AN ANTIOXIDANT AUTHORITY

Meet Joe A. Vinson, Ph.D., from the University of Scranton in Pennsylvania, researcher and author of stacks of studies, including some on the healing compounds in superfoods. While he does say the *superfoods* term sometimes is not science based, he acknowledges the nutrient-dense, wholesome foods that are believed to be healthy choices. And, if he was marooned on an island, can you guess what superfoods he'd choose for survival? Read on—you may be pleasantly surprised!

Q: *Ancient grains such as oats are known to be healthful. Why do ancient grains make the typical superfoods list?*

A: Oats are highest in polyphenols [plant-based micronutrients that might help lower your odds of developing cancer or heart disease] and antioxidants among all the flours and also the highest on the ready-to-eat breakfast cereals.

Q: *Potatoes (especially fast-food-chain fried ones) have been given a bad rap. Why do you feel we should include them in moderation in our diet?*

A: Potatoes eaten with the skin will provide the most fiber, nutrients, and polyphenols. Purple potatoes have significantly more polyphenols than white potatoes. [These little super potatoes come from South America. Available year-round, they contain a four-fold amount of antioxidants compared with Russet potatoes. Golf ball–size, they're used in salads and soups, and available in supermarkets.]

Q: *Berries (such as blueberries) get a lot of credit in superfood literature. But what about cranberries and strawberries? Please tell me why these other berries are nutritious, too. Aren't cranberries as rich in antioxidants as blueberries?*

A: Each berry has a different spectrum of polyphenols, and we need to get as many and as much polyphenols in our diet as possible for maximum health benefits.

Q: *Spinach and kale—two touted health foods. Mixing the two make our food more flavorful. Are these leafy greens (washed to rid of pesticides) rich in antioxidants? Do you consider them important in a healthiest foods list?*

A: Leafy vegetables are not particularly high in polyphenols and antioxidants, but again, we need a spectrum of polyphenols in our diet and as much fiber as possible.

Q: *If you were stranded on an island and could have five foods to eat for two weeks (you get water), what would you eat, and briefly share why these are your choices.*

A: Nuts, peanut butter, orange juice, wine, and whole-grain crackers (to put the peanut butter on). The solid foods are filling and tasty. The liquids contain polyphenols and taste good, too, and the orange juice provides vitamin C.

SUPERFOODS TIDBITS TO CHEW ON

As medical researchers continue to make breakthrough discoveries about disease-fighting antioxidants, research and marketing companies keep track of food trends, year after year. Also, projections are doled out on how long which superfoods will stay in demand or if they're just a whim that'll fade. Here, take a look at the consensus, and you can make your own forecast for the growth of superfoods in the future.

- The term *superfood* has become a buzzword in the language of food and health. Some nutritionists and medical doctors shun the word because they claim there is lack of scientific evidence to back the praise for some foods.
- Producers and marketers of superfoods highlight this term to add extra value in order to sell their products. Foods that are often sold as superfoods include ancient grains, salad mixes, seeds, and seaweeds.
- Nutritionists point out a trend of "mindful eating," a slower and more thoughtful approach to eating.
- More than half of consumers in a poll will choose to "eat clean" by looking to eat foods that are less processed and more whole foods such as vegetables, fruits, and ancient grains, as well as plant-based proteins like nuts and seeds.
- Top superfoods have included ancient grains, avocados, coconut products, exotic fruits, green tea, kale, nuts, seeds, salmon, and fermented foods like yogurt.

My goal includes focusing on common superfoods that may not surprise you, but adding new findings, twists, and turns for each one that will open your eyes. I'm also combining twentieth-century favorite comfort dishes with new superfoods. Read: You'll be discovering unprocessed superfoods that have super flavor and versatility—and are easy to find at the local supermarket. That means no treks to find obscure foods. It's time. It's time to get real food without bells and whistles.

WHAT'S SO SUPER ABOUT SUPERFOODS?

Enter superfoods. The thing is (despite skeptical doctors and nutritionists who insist superfoods are a marketing tool to lure consumers to buy an item, like the aphrodisiac maca or bottled green drinks) some down-to-earth foods are nutrient dense and super! And there is a new school of food wizards who will tell you superfoods are real, with an abundance of nutrients and can be combined in a balanced diet regime and/or used topically for beauty.

Yes, eating superfoods can be super. I'm dishing up good, clean eating—whole, natural foods, low in sugar, salt, and fat, including fruits, vegetables, dairy, nuts, fish, and whole grains. Also, the superfoods in this book are not just about clean foods, but also your enjoyment of both the taste and benefits of "semiclean" functional foods, such as the "new" superfoods gelato and shellfish, which are healthiest when eaten in moderation.

The majority of the doctors I've interviewed during the past three decades praised the healing powers of nutrient-dense "power foods" (such as fruits, vegetables, eggs, fish and poultry). Both conventional and holistic medical experts shared personal experiences about how exactly these foods helped them and/or their patients lose unwanted weight and fight chronic ailments, even heart disease.

But back in those days we didn't say "superfood"; instead, phrases to describe the healthiest foods included *healing*, *cancer-fighting*, *pound-pairing*, *miracle*, and *wonder* foods. And wonderful they can be, so wonderful the term *superfoods* is now a household word and not just jargon for health nuts. In fact, while supplements played a big role in the early twentieth century, a nutrient-dense diet seems to be more in demand unless there is a lack of a certain mineral or vitamin in an individual's diet.

Here, take a look at some of the good-for-you antioxidants, polyphenols, minerals, and vitamins found in superfoods that may help stave off cellular damage, and you'll begin to get why the superfood craze is not just a fad—it is here to stay.

SUPER HEALTH-BOOSTING NUTRIENTS IN SUPERFOODS

Superfoods Group	Nutrient Category	What Superfoods Can Do
Vegetables, super-fruits	Carotenoids	Powerful disease fighters that may lower risk of cancer, heart disease
Supergrains	Dietary fiber	Lower the risk of developing cancer, heart disease, diabetes
Nuts	Fatty acids, protein	Lower the risk of developing heart disease, boost the immune system
Vegetables, super-fruits	Flavonoids	Disease fighters that may help to lower the risk of developing cancer, heart disease
Ancient grains, eggs, nuts, vegetables	Minerals	May reduce high blood pressure, lower risk of chronic ailments
Dairy, nuts, vegetables	Phytoestrogens	May lower risk of heart disease, enhance immune system
Dairy, fish, poultry, seeds, superfruits	Vitamins	Boost immune system, lower risk of heart disease

So, now that you understand my desire to dish up superfoods (especially favorite foods that you can find in your local supermarket), why not take a break and digest the premise of superfoods and how they can be healing. Go ahead—whip up a fruit juice beverage to get in the mood for discovering clean food that'll help you feel good and energized.

Super Detoxifying Pure Cleanse

❖ ❖ ❖

It's time to enjoy a simple, natural beverage to savor while you indulge in the following pages about superfoods and how they can help you feel super! This recipe is health spa–inspired and served to spa goers.

1¾ *cups green apples*
1 *cup guava (or use fresh berries)*

Juice all of the ingredients, then pour into a glass and serve immediately.

Makes 1 serving.
(Courtesy: Chiva-Som International Health Resort)

In this book, I will show you how classic favorite foods can be the new superfoods and how adding them to your diet today can bring you brighter tomorrows. But many people, perhaps you, will not want to reap the benefits of all superfoods. So, if you don't like one or are allergic to it, there are substitutes. You can use superfoods in other amazing ways, too. I've included dozens of recipes for eating as well as some to use topically as household cleaners, beauty aids, and home cures.

But first, let's go way, way back into the past. Going back to basic superfoods feels like I'm a time traveler revisiting places I've been and places I've loved and places I aspire to go to in the future. And enjoying favorite functional foods is part of the package. Take a journey with me to discover the history of superfoods and how foods with healing powers are nature's medicine.

SUPER-IOR HEALING SUPERFOODS FOR THOUGHT

Research in the latter part of the twentieth century and the early twenty-first century shows that nutrient-dense, functional foods, which come from nature, produce a diet that can protect your health—and may help you to:

✓ Enhance your immune system
✓ Fight fat
✓ Lower your blood pressure
✓ Lower the risk of heart disease
✓ Lower the risk of developing cancer
✓ Slow the aging process and add years to your life

History of Healing Foods

*The doctor of the future will no longer treat the
human frame with drugs, but rather will cure and
prevent disease with nutrition.*
—THOMAS EDISON

My first real-life superfoods meal I recall was a peanut butter and
strawberry jam sandwich when I was two years old in Northern
California—a region rich in superfoods berries and nuts. By the seventies, the utopia-like orchards and groves mutated into the urban
sprawl of Silicon Valley. But back in the fifties, I was the middle child
of three, with a mom and dad, living in a neighborhood of suburban
tract homes with sidewalks, mowed lawns, and nearby schools and
malls. We were enveloped by Garden of Eve–like gardens and a myriad
of roadside produce stands on the outskirts of town, on the route to
Central California, the heart of superfoods.

One Thanksgiving (before urbanization) I helped my mom cook
and bake in the kitchen. I scrutinized her savvy moves like viewing
Julia Child on TV. My mother was on duty to craft a feast (like that autumn New England first harvest feast shared by the Pilgrims and
Indians). The superfoods menu included turkey, cranberries, leafy
greens, sweet potatoes, and pecan pie. By afternoon the table spread in
our minimalist-decorated dining room was a *Moveable Feast* event.

After eating a bit of each superfood (except ignoring the sweet potatoes, which weren't sweet to my unsophisticated palate), I was excused from the table. My goal was to escape to the cozy family room and play with Casey, our Dalmatian. Using turkey tidbits to teach him tricks was fun until I heard the familiar words from my mom: "We're taking a box of food to the girls."

This trip was an adventure, driving through downtown, passing by the Doggie Diner and Bob's Big Boy Restaurant, to give the gift of real food to my mother's two friends, Florence and Dorothy (who resembled the matriarch Sophia Petrillo in TV's *The Golden Girls*). Both elderly widows were delighted to receive superfood care packages. Going home while listening to KLIV radio pop songs, there was a superb feeling to know we delivered a turkey dinner like the Thanksgiving feast shared centuries ago instead of fast food. Praising real food—not processed glop in a bag—is going back to my roots. But nature's superfoods go further back in time than when I was a kid. Let's take a peek at when clean food was shared way, way back during the early-man era.

THE STONE AGE

Welcome to the Paleo diet, also known as the caveman diet. Back-to-nature foods were hunted and gathered during Paleolithic times. The eats included fish, nuts, leafy greens, vegetables, and seeds—the same edibles in superfoods lists in the modern day. Some medical and diet researchers believe that while the ancient foods diet without dairy has a good ratio of good and bad fats, the lack of calcium is not a good thing. But I've learned diets, like health, are a controversial topic—past and present.

CENTURIES OF SUPERFOODS

In other books about superfoods, you will not easily find a food time line, especially for the specific word *superfood*,—but this doesn't mean that superfoods were nonexistent. Indeed, superfoods existed since the beginning of time!

So, I went to work and pieced a time line together from food historians, century by century, and discovered which foods and food trends were popular. It's interesting to see how nature's finest foods were eaten in the earlier centuries, then before the turn of the twentieth century. What is surprising is what happens in the mid-1900s and how we've almost come full circle in the present day. Read on.

1500s: Medieval times were challenging since all superfruits and vegetables were cooked because of the belief that they carried disease if eaten raw. Peasants kept cows, so eating cheese, another touted super-food, was part of their diet.

1600s: The English diet included greens, such as spinach, as well as fresh fruit and nuts—all known superfoods from the caveman era to the twenty-first century—that were foraged from the wild.

1700s: The New England colonists ate superfoods, including potatoes, oats, and turkey, and indulged in imported cheese from Europe. In the classic food scene in the film *Tom Jones*—based on Henry Fielding's eighteenth-century novel *The History of Tom Jones, a Foundling*—superfoods, including chicken, shellfish, and apples, were savored during a delectable table feast.

1800s: During the nineteenth century, most people lived on farms. During harvest time, superfoods could be plentiful. Farmers made cheese from milks their cows provided and chickens gave eggs. Fresh vegetables were eaten only in season. In the Midwest, potatoes were a staple, with citrus fruits in the South, and apples were plentiful in the fall. Back in England, oats, an ancient supergrain, played a role in the Charles Dickens classic *Oliver Twist* when the boy begged for more gruel, a nineteenth-century staple (a mix of boiled oatmeal and butter).

THE TWENTIETH-CENTURY SUPERFOODS PARADE

At the turn of the twentieth century, the United Fruit Company got testimonials from medical doctors and nutritionists to tout the banana as a superfood. In the 1900s, osteopaths pointed out that the sacred superfruit was sealed by nature in a practically germ-free package.

After World War II, the fifties baby boom hit and the economy was good. This, in turn, spawned the popularity of eating out at restaurants and then fast-food outlets. Also, meat and potatoes were more in vogue than fresh fruit and vegetables. Processed frozen foods gained momentum thanks to the luxury of a freezer.

Superfoods existed, but often they were not sold or eaten in their natural state. Overcooking vegetables in soups and stews was not unheard of, and fried foods, whether it be chicken or onion rings, took the super out of foods fast.

I lived through the transformation of food into superfoods during the 1960s hippie era, a time of eating the strict "macrobiotic" whole foods, and then superfruit juice fasting in the seventies. Not to forget the health foods, which included bean sprouts, salads, yogurt, and whole-grain foods such as brown rice. It was clean food eating but not exactly mainstream; these superfoods drew in the health-conscious people or the health nuts who frequented health food stores. The superfood storm had not yet hit mainstream America.

While both foraging berries, nuts, and seeds and hunting game and fishing by the cavemen and eating the fresh fare from farms in the nineteenth century seem to be the healthiest eating styles, health food trends and health foods gained popularity in the 1900s.

But the top 20 superfoods I've selected have held a steady position around the world, century by century. It's the simple, back-to-nature foods that have become tagged health foods or superfoods. No fads—just real, clean food for your mind, body, and spirit.

NEW SUPERFOODS

Eating twentieth-century and twenty-first-century foods is a bit mind-boggling. It's a mix of down-to-earth real food that we're turning back to, much like foods in the seventies. I've experienced different waves of food trends—some healthy, some not healthy. But as time passes, people in the food industry are learning what is better for our overall health and well-being. It turns out, simple is better, and going back to nature is best.

Eating a variety of superfood groups is an ongoing theme in the *Healing Powers* series, and *The Healing Powers of Superfoods* is no exception. As Will Clower, Ph.D., the C.E.O. and go-to person at

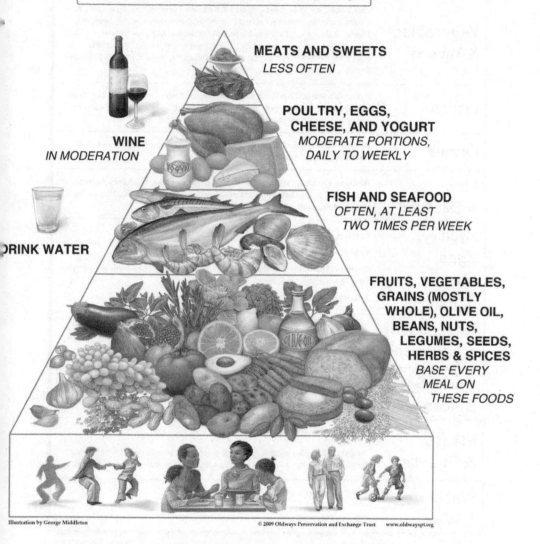

Mediterranean Diet Pyramid
A contemporary approach to delicious, healthy eating

MEATS AND SWEETS
LESS OFTEN

**POULTRY, EGGS,
CHEESE, AND YOGURT**
*MODERATE PORTIONS,
DAILY TO WEEKLY*

WINE
IN MODERATION

FISH AND SEAFOOD
*OFTEN, AT LEAST
TWO TIMES PER WEEK*

DRINK WATER

**FRUITS, VEGETABLES,
GRAINS (MOSTLY
WHOLE), OLIVE OIL,
BEANS, NUTS,
LEGUMES, SEEDS,
HERBS & SPICES**
*BASE EVERY
MEAL ON
THESE FOODS*

BE PHYSICALLY ACTIVE; ENJOY MEALS WITH OTHERS

Mediterranean Wellness, pointed out in the foreword, the Mediterranean diet includes my top favorite picks. In an A–Z order, common foods of the groups are: cheese and yogurt, eggs, fruits, fish and seafood, grains, meats and sweets, nuts, poultry, seeds, vegetables, water, and wine.

Common Foods and Flavors of the Mediterranean Diet Pyramid

Vegetables & Tubers	Artichokes, Arugula, Beets, Broccoli, Brussels Sprouts, Cabbage, Carrots, Celery, Celeriac, Chicory, Collard Cucumber, Dandelion Greens, Eggplant, Fennel, Kale, Leeks, Lettuce, Mache, Mushrooms, Mustard Greens, Nettles, Okra, Onions (red, sweet, white), Peas, Peppers, Potatoes, Pumpkin, Purslane, Radishes, Rutabega, Scallions, Shallots, Spinach, Sweet Potatoes, Turnips, Zucchini
Fruits	Avocados, Apples, Apricots, Cherries, Clementines, Dates, Figs, Grapefruit, Grapes, Lemons, Oranges, Melons, Nectarines, Olives, Peaches, Pears, Pomegranates, Strawberries, Tangerines, Tomatoes
Grains	Breads, Barley, Buckwheat, Bulgur, Couscous, Durum, Farro, Millet, Oats, Polenta, Rice, Wheatberries
Fish & Seafood	Abalone, Cockles, Clams, Crab, Eel, Flounder, Lobster, Mackerel, Mussels, Octopus, Oysters, Salmon, Sardines, Sea Bass, Shrimp, Squid, Tilapia, Tuna, Whelk, Yellowtail
Poultry, Eggs, Cheese, & Yogurt	Chicken, Duck, Guinea Fowl Eggs (Chicken, Quail, and Duck) Cheeses (Examples Include: Brie, Chevre, Corvo, Feta, Haloumi, Manchego, Parmigiano-Reggiano, Pecorino, Ricotta) Yogurt, Greek Yogurt
Nuts, Seeds, & Legumes	Almonds, Beans (Cannellini, Chickpeas, Fava, Kidney, Green), Cashews, Hazelnuts, Lentils, Pine Nuts, Pistachios, Sesame Seeds (Tahini), Split Peas, Walnuts
Herbs & Spices	Anise, Basil, Bay Leaf, Chiles, Clove, Cumin, Fennel, Garlic, Lavender, Marjoram, Mint, Oregano, Parsley, Pepper, Pul Biber, Rosemary, Sage, Savory, Sumac, Tarragon, Thyme, Za'atar
Meats & Sweets	Pork, Beef, Lamb, Mutton, Goat Sweets (Examples include: Baklava, Biscotti, Crème Caramel, Chocolate, Gelato, Fruit Tarts, Kunefe, Lokum, Mousse Au Chocolat, Sorbet, Tiramisu)
Water & Wine	Drink Plenty of Water Wine in Moderation

When I chose *my* favorite superfoods (many are the same choices in a random poll I took by asking, "If you were stranded on an island for two weeks, what five foods would you choose for survival?"), I was surprised that many of my picks were also included in the Oldways Mediterranean Diet Pyramid. Take a look at the Mediterranean foods and you'll discover everything you need to know about the top 20 I include in the following chapters.

OTHER PAST MEDICAL USES OF SUPERFOODS

The uses of healing foods with superpowers trace back to ancient history. Historical references to superfoods are backed up by the consensus of functional food proponents. In all fairness, a past milestone shouldn't be attributed to one source, especially if it happened centuries ago. Legends reveal that humankind may have known that superfoods held healing powers thousands of years ago.

Historical	Uses	Method/Superfood
Pre-*Homo* species	Gathered fruits and seeds to eat raw	Food
Paleolithic era peoples	Berries, fruits nuts, seeds, fish, meat	Food
Neolithic era peoples	Ancient grains	Food
Aztecs	Chia seeds	Food
Ancient Romans	Berries	Alleviated symptoms of melancholy, fainting
American Indians	Berries	Medicinal purposes
Civil War soldiers	Berry beverage	Improved health

OTHER SUPERFOOD MILESTONES OF THE TWENTIETH AND TWENTY-FIRST CENTURIES

Superfood historians agree on the time frame in which nutrient-rich foods made their mark around the globe. Here are a few highlights, showing when the healing powers of functional foods made their debut in the mainstream media and everyday peoples' lives.

MODERN-DAY SUPERFOODS TIME LINE

Decade	What Happened	What It Did
1970s	Health and fitness guru Adelle Davis's books make splash	Promoted organic foods movement
1980s	Ancient Harvest company was first to bring quinoa to United States	Created awareness of ancient grains
1990s	1. Mattson's VP Innovation noted blueberries ignited the superfood trend	Created demand to buy and eat berries
	2. Antioxidant-rich foods noted in media	Increased consumer awareness
Early 2000s	Quinoa jumped on the touted superfood bandwagon	Media/consumer demand soars
2000s	1. Sambazon Superfruit Smoothies supercharged with vitamins	Boosted smoothie trend
	2. Kale, seaweed, superfruits, and other superfood "flavors of the year" sprout	Media/health-conscious consumers buy into superfoods
2003	Superfood term makes news; release of bestseller Super-Foods Rx	Mainstream choose superfoods
2005	Thousands of new products tout berries as superfruits	Demand for berries soars
2011–15	Food/beverage products containing the terms superfood, superfruit, and supergrain double	Consumer superfood awareness grows

As you can see, superfoods have been noticed for good reason as healing foods from ancient times to the present day, in the United States and around the globe. These unforgettable historical highlights are to show you how superfoods are not just a fad or marketing tool for food items. Nature's foods have been used for food and medicinal purposes and go back to the beginning of time. Yes, the word *superfoods* may be a "new age" term, but the concept is from the beginning of time and these favorite foods are pillars in a healthful diet.

Super Brain-Enhancing Grilled Salmon with Almonds

In the top 20 superfoods spotlighted in this book, I include shellfish instead of wild salmon (another popular superfood) because it deserves recognition, too. This entrée recipe, however, grabbed my attention because it does include many of my picks and contains olive oil and vinegar—two ancient superfoods that you'll see like recurring characters in *The Healing Powers of Superfoods*. Also, while I dish up vegan vegetarian entrees, raw foods, fresh salads, smoothies, and soups, my favorite foods also include fish—and that includes salmon.

Salt and pepper, to taste
4 salmon steaks
4 tablespoons curry powder
2 tablespoons almond or olive oil
1½ cups mixed lettuce greens
1 small papaya
¼ medium red onion
1 tomato
10 sprigs coriander
4 tablespoons almond oil (for dressing)
2 tablespoons raspberry vinegar
⅓ cup natural California almonds, coarsely chopped

Salt and pepper the salmon steaks, then rub with curry powder. Grease steaks with almond or olive oil and set aside. Wash lettuce. Peel papaya, cut in halves, and core with a spoon. Cut papaya in quarters; keep a few slices for decoration and dice the rest. Peel onion and cut into fine slices. Dice tomato and chop coriander. Toss diced papaya, onion, tomato, and coriander with lettuce. Marinate salad mixture with almond oil and raspberry vinegar. Grill steaks in a pan on both sides 3–5 minutes.

Serve on salad. Sprinkle with chopped almonds and decorate with papaya slices.

Makes 4 servings.
(Courtesy: *Almonds Are in the Kitchen,* Almond Board of California)

In the next chapter, you'll be departing the historical world of healing foods as I take you into the twenty-first century. While you'll get a taste of the twentieth-century classic favorite foods, I'm changing it up to give you a healthy mix of superfoods gone both crazy-comforting and healthy.

SUPER-IOR HEALING SUPERFOODS FOR THOUGHT

✓ Functional foods can be traced back to ancient times, from the biblical era to caveman days, when nature's finest foods were eaten for survival and their medicinal remedies were praised.
✓ Superfoods were recognized for their healing powers by the Romans, Egyptians, and Aztecs, and eventually made a splash around the world.
✓ By the fifteenth century, superfoods were used by Europeans (especially royalty, but peasants, too), who used healthful foods for foodstuffs and medicinal uses.
✓ In the eighteenth century, superfoods had made their way to North America and continued to expand to the northeast and across the continent. The versatile foods were used to help heal the mind, body, and spirit.
✓ The nineteenth and twentieth centuries experienced controversy about specific superfoods—such that the health virtues of eggs, fatty foods, and dairy foods were ignored. But nowadays, these forbidden foods are accepted as healthy fare (eaten in moderation).
✓ Today, superfoods are used as food and beverages, in weight loss programs, in beauty and cleaning products, and as home cures (topically and eaten) by people in the United States and around the globe.

PART 2

TOP 20 SUPERFOODS

Apples

It is remarkable how closely the history of the apple tree is connected with that of man.
—Henry David Thoreau, Wild Fruits:
Thoreau's Rediscovered Last Manuscript

While my first memory of superfoods is peanut butter and strawberry jam, apples are the number-one superstar food for me as an adult with the heart of a kid. Autumn and winter still make me feel warm and fuzzy when I recall the suburban vibe, with yards chock-full of fruit trees and their fruits, including apples, especially during holiday baking. A variety of types of apples have made it into my life year-round. The Granny Smith tart, green apples take me back to childhood and one specific Sunday winter morning.

As a constant fan of my mom's baking finesse, I was invited by her one overcast Christmas school break to help make a Waldorf salad. My mom, like a hybrid of the twentieth-first-century Food Network celebrity chefs like Pioneer Woman and Barefoot Contessa, set out superfoods on the salmon-colored-tile kitchen countertop. My eyes opened wide as I sized up the fresh green and red apples, celery stalks, green grapes, and chopped walnuts—and mayonnaise. My mother (a suburbanite Elizabeth Taylor look-alike) went to work chopping apples. I didn't want to use the mini-sized white marshmallows, which I suggested to exclude and keep for cocoa. My mom, a traditionalist, said, "Follow instructions." She told me her conventional salad had roots all the way back to 1896 and the Waldorf Hotel. When it was served as a side dish for dinner, I rebelled and picked out the white squishy balls, one by one.

Years later, my Waldorf salad, not my mother's recipe, got a makeover with a superfoods twist. I use Greek yogurt instead of mayonnaise, fresh lemon (not the juice out of a bottle), and raw, local honey instead of marshmallows. The fruit salad is better the new way, but I understand my mom, who liked to follow tradition and use recipes from Irma S. Rombauer's *Joy of Cooking*, a bible for cooking in the twentieth century (the Waldorf salad called for mayo). But apples (unlike sweeteners) are a superfruit in recipes that do not change throughout time.

THE HISTORY OF APPLES

Meet the apple tree (*Malus pumila*). If you look back in time, you'll find artwork showing Adam and Eve in the Garden of Eden with the forbidden fruit—a red apple. Apples were historically found around the globe, and apple varieties from Central Asia and Europe were brought to North America by European colonists. By the seventeenth century, the first apple orchard was planted in Boston by Reverend William Blaxton. In the 1800s and early 1900s, the demand for apples grew in the United States.

By the twentieth century, Washington State joined the apple bandwagon, and the Pacific Northwest state is one of the leading states for growing the superfruit. In the twenty-first century, apples continue to be in demand, and apple picking on farms is a popular trend. (There is more of a selection in the fall.)

Ode to Johnny Appleseed

One of America's favored legends, told by both apple farmers and food historians, is the story of a folk hero and pioneer farmer in the nineteenth century. Legend tells it the man's real name was John Chapman, from Leominster, Massachusetts. His dream was for the land to produce so many apples that no one would ever go hungry.

A businessman ahead of this time, Chapman traveled new frontiers, developing nurseries of apple trees. For decades he journeyed through the Midwest. His mission was planting apple seeds. He also tended to apple orchards as well as other fruit plants. He believed God wanted him to tour solo and plant seeds to grow apple trees for humanity. And he did just that.

Super Nutrients

Apples (unlike some other superfruits that are difficult to find in the winter months) are readily available year-round (but not all varieties) and are a nutritious and popular fruit. This favorite fruit is versatile in cooking and baking, it appeals to people of all ages, and its nutrients are amazing—with some surprises.

Eating an apple a day may mean fewer doctors to pay, according to the ancient proverb and even twenty-first-century medical studies, which I discovered while researching the use of apples in apple cider vinegar in Vinegarland for my book *The Healing Powers of Vinegar*. True, those little green apples (red and yellow ones, too) don't contain tons of good-for-you vitamins and minerals (similar to when you look at the nutrition label of apple cider vinegar) but they are good apples because they contain surprise ingredients.

Yes, apples are a superfood with disease-fighting antioxidants and are something to write home about. Apples are low in calories, fat-free, and don't have cholesterol or sodium; they're a dieter's best friend. But there's much more! Here's why that fresh, crisp apple you like to bite into, sprinkle in salads, add to smoothies, and bake into pies, scones, and tarts (and sip as apple juice) is a super-duper superfood that dishes healing powers.

HEALTH BENEFITS OF APPLES

The dietary fiber, for starters, found in an apple is soluble fiber found in the fruit's pectin, and it may be helpful in lowering levels of the "bad" blood cholesterol called low-density lipoprotein (LDL). High levels of this type of cholesterol are linked to possible heart disease and may increase the odds of heart attack or stroke due to plaque that can clog arteries. (This topic bored me when I was young and felt invincible; but now cholesterol-friendly foods are my friends for my heart's sake.)

Also, apples are a good source of potassium, which may help provide protection against strokes. And like most other superfruits (such as ones with skins, like apricots, grapes, pears, and plums), their low sodium content is good for keeping blood pressure numbers in check. But there's more to the almighty apple that will make you want to have an apple tree in your yard or go apple picking at a farm.

Stacks and stacks of studies show that apples contain disease-fighting antioxidants, such as flavonoids, that may lower the risk of developing heart disease and certain cancers. Apples rank number two in having the highest level of antioxidant activity of any other superfruit—except for the little red, round tart cranberry.[1]

The efficacy of prescribing an apple a day instead of statins (cholesterol-lowering drugs) was discovered in one study by a research group at Oxford University in the United Kingdom. The researchers based their intriguing findings on mathematical model calculations (not lab rats). The scientists' results, published in the *British Medical Journal*, show that prescribing an apple a day to adults aged fifty-plus could result in 8,500 fewer heart attacks and strokes each year in the United Kingdom—results similar to those of statins, without the side effects.[2]

What's more, according to findings, some types of apples rank higher on the superfood list. Apples are all healthful, but it seems a few may contain more disease-fighting powers from polyphenol antioxidants. Using a past study of different apples, researchers published a list of the apples ranking high in antioxidants in *Journal of Food Science* that may surprise you. The crabapple (small wild apples), Ida red, Red Delicious, Honey Crisp, and Granny Smith are the top apple winners you may want to favor, according to the researchers.[3]

Studies are plentiful on apples and health. Scientists at the Institute of Food Research conducted a study published in *Molecular Nutrition & Food Research* that reveals more good news for apple lovers. Some compounds like polyphenols in both green tea and apples inhibit a key molecule called VEGF, in the body which can contribute to diseases such as cancer and heart attacks. This may explain why polyphenol-rich foods lower the risk of developing chronic diseases, keeping you healthier, and perhaps that's why apples may help keep the doctor at bay longer, too.[4]

Super Heart-Healthy Cinna-Apple Smoothie

❖ ❖ ❖

Most of the smoothies I share with you include easy-to-find, simple superfoods available at your local supermarket. This Cinna-Apple Smoothie, however, does contain a few somewhat uncommon ingredients, including cran-water, flaxseed oil, flaxseeds (flax is rich in alpha-linolenic acid, a kind of omega-3 fatty acid that may help lower your risk of developing heart disease), powdered probiotic (which are living bacteria and yeasts that provide health benefits, especially for the digestive system) and powdered whey protein. If you prefer, substitute powdered probiotic with yogurt, use flaxseeds but not oil, and try a bit of nut butter instead of powdered whey protein. These superfood health ingredients can be found at a health food store. It's a nutrient-dense smoothie for no-nonsense health nuts.[5]

8 ounces purified water
    or cran-water
1 scoop powdered whey
    protein (Fat Flush)
1 scoop powdered pro-
    biotic
1 tablespoon flaxseed oil
1 tablespoon ground
    flaxseeds

1 small organic apple,
    peeled and cut into
    chunks
½ teaspoon Ceylon cinna-
    mon, or to taste
Ice cubes (optional)

Combine water, powders, flaxseed oil and seeds, apple, cinnamon, and ice in blender until smooth.

Makes 1 serving.
(Courtesy: Ann Louise Gittleman, Ph.D., C.N.S.)

Now that you're aware of superpowers of the apple, I'll show you in Chapter 4 how berries—another sweet superfood used since the Stone Age era, continue to get a smile from medical doctors and researchers, nutritionists, consumers—and me. It's the pureness of wild berries that won my taste buds as a kid, and this superfruit may be one of your favorite superfoods, too. While blueberries are the touted number-one superfood, I'm branching out—no need to neglect their counterparts.

SUPER-IOR HEALING SUPERFOODS FOR THOUGHT

✓ Apples may help lower the risk of developing cancers, reduce bad cholesterol, boost immunity, and much more.
✓ All types of apples and their superpowers are acknowledged around the world as healing medicines. But some varieties contain more disease-fighting antioxidants than others.
✓ Apples are a dieter's best friend because they are low in calories and contain no fat, no sodium, and no cholesterol.
✓ And apples contain dietary fiber that is heart-healthy and antioxidants that may help lower the risk of heart disease and cancer.

4

Berries (and Avocados)

Two lovely berries moulded on one stem;
So with two seeming bodies, but one heart.
—WILLIAM SHAKESPEARE, *Midsummer's Night's Dream*

At age twelve, I was an adventurous kid drawn to nature's superfoods and the great outdoors. One cloudy afternoon, a girlfriend and I hiked to the Los Gatos foothills, where grass wasn't manicured and horses ran free. Trespassing on pristine grounds and picking wild red berries off plants was an exciting novelty until it began to pour down rain. The thrill of the exploration was worth getting soaked. But once we were home the escapade hadn't even started.

I took a hot shower and cleaned off the mud on my body. Later, at night, I scratched my cheek, arms, and legs because for some unknown reason they itched. By morning when I awoke, red bumps and blisters were visible on my face. "Poison oak," my mother announced after I told her where I had gone the day before. I blamed it on that reddish-colored plant that my wilderness companion had pointed out to me; we had been surrounded by the toxic bushes. By dinnertime my face was red, and one of my puffy and painful eyelids was swollen shut. My two siblings chanted "Cyclops," insinuating I looked like the spooky one-eyed creature in mythology. I ran into my bedroom, onto the bed, and hid underneath the covers.

Later, my mom consoled me. She sat on the bed and said, "Ignore your brother and sister." She handed me a bowl of fresh, store-bought, red, juicy berries that were cold and comforting as she told me a story about the Greeks and Romans. Evidently, they used the wild strawberry plant for medicinal powers. I savored the historically therapeutic berries, believing the blisters and bumps would heal in time. And they did.

THE HISTORY OF BERRIES

As noted in the previous chapter, it's known that berries have been a valued food source for humans and other primates since the beginning of agriculture back to the prehistoric era. This versatile superfruit—and super clean food—a seasonal staple for hunters and gatherers for centuries—was not taken for granted. Wild berry foraging has been popular in the past centuries and still is in the present day in both Europe and North America.

Berry experts and food historians agree that the favorite blackberry and much-loved raspberry have been enjoyed in both their raw forms and in cuisine since the seventeenth century, whereas the blueberry and cranberry made their debut as favored foods after that. And the juicy red strawberry, the most popular berry in the twenty-first century, is a standout in dishes, including savory salads and sweet desserts.

Legend of the Super Miracle Berry

As the story goes, the sacred blueberry was gathered and used by Native Americans for centuries before European colonists arrived. The Native Americans believed that the little, vibrant-colored blueberries were sent by the Great Spirit during a great famine to relieve the hunger of their children. Indians knew blueberries were healthful, so they believed they were a miracle berry that was a godsend to mankind—one of the first superfoods but without the "super" label.[1]

SUPER NUTRIENTS

While berries are known as past and present superfruits, it's not just the blueberry that deserves credit for its nutritional perks. Sure, antioxidant-rich acai berries and goji berries are good berries, but seriously, do you love these varieties more than classic vitamin C–rich favorites like scrumptious blackberries in a cobbler, cranberry scones, raspberries in a jam, and strawberry gelato?

Unless you're a serious, purist foodie on the hunt for exotic superfoods (often difficult to find in your local supermarket), it's likely that common but also nutritious berries are your true friends (not the strange newbies). Berries are touted for their dietary fiber, the water-soluble type called pectin.

Stacks of research studies show that this fabulous fiber helps lower unhealthy blood cholesterol levels by soaking up cholesterol by-products in the intestinal tract and carrying them out of the body. Not only are berries heart-healthy wonders, but one cup of berries also dishes up about half of your RDA for vitamin C—the immune-boosting nutrient to keep you healthy year-round.[2]

Blackberry (*Rubus*): A delicious berry rich in dietary fiber, vitamin C, and vitamin K. A half cup is a mere 43 calories. The blackberry is rich in antioxidants, including carotenoids, ellagitannins, and ellagic acid. A summertime favorite, but can be found year-round in different forms (dried and frozen).

Cranberry (*Vaccinium*): Touted as another superfruit, this little berry is also packed with immune-boosting vitamin C, dietary fiber, manganese, and heart-healthy flavonoids. Fresh cranberries seem to get noticed during autumn and winter as well as the holiday season—then they're forgotten.

Raspberry (*Rubus idaeus*): This little berry—both sweet and tart varieties—turns out to be a favorite of berry lovers. At a bit more than 50 calories and six grams of fiber per cup, it's a super anticancer and heart-healthy fruit. Also, it can do much more, from helping relieve digestion ailments to aiding in weight loss—which are discussed later on in chapters dishing on home cures and weight loss.

Strawberry (*Fragaria*): This is another sweet, juicy fruit chock-full in vitamin C. It also contains two flavonoids, quercetin and kaempferol, which may help keep blood platelets from clumping together and help lower the risk of heart disease.[3])

HEALTH BENEFITS OF BERRIES

Not unlike apples, for berries, it's not just the fiber, the vitamin C, and the diet-friendly traits that are super, it's also the super disease-fighting antioxidant power that makes berries a superfood. So there are extra heart-health merits to berries thanks to their powerful phytochemicals, such as catechins, which have been shown to inhibit the buildup of cholesterol and lower levels of cholesterol (the sticky plaque that can clog your arteries and lead to heart attacks and strokes).

Like other antioxidant-rich superfoods, berries can and do provide protection for both your heart and immune system, which also means berries may help you lower the risk of developing a cold, flu, or even cancer. That means you can savor your favorite berries for their healing powers by eating more rather than less. Mix them up in cereals, salads and smoothies.

Surprisingly, the blueberry isn't the most popular. In a favorite-berry poll I took, the blackberry, raspberry, and strawberry have devoted followers. But the cranberry, my latest berry love, with its super nutrients, versatility, and healing powers, is in the limelight more.

Cranberry Love

Cranberries were an unknown pleasure to author and olive oil expert Judy Ridgeway, based in the United Kingdom, until she tasted cranberry sauce at an American friend's Thanksgiving dinner. "I was an instant convert and started to think about how to use them in my own cooking," she recalls. Later, the cranberry fan discovered the berries were difficult to find in the UK marketplace, but as time passed she learned cranberries are can be found either fresh in season, or frozen or dried throughout the year. Here is the cranberry lover's favorite superfoods berry and cheese dip, and her words for me and you to share its deliciousness.

Cheese and Cranberry Dip

❖ ❖ ❖

This dip helps to get the party going. It looks stunning served in a large bowl, surrounded by crackers, vegetable crudités, and corn chips for dunking. Invite everyone to help themselves. The recipe uses dried cranberries. These are a useful standby to have in the cupboard; however, they do not have quite the item in content of the fresh fruit. If the dried berries are too dried out, soak them by dunking them for one hour in hot water or overnight in cold water.

A big chunk of Brie (approximately 1 pound)
1 fresh garlic clove, crushed
1 slosh of wine
1 handful of dried cranberries

Make a "bowl" shape from tinfoil and place the cheese inside. Toss the ingredients over the top artistically and close the top of the tinfoil bowl so that it covers the contents completely. Place the whole parcel on a baking tray to catch any drips. Bake in a medium-heated oven 10–15 minutes, until the cheese is gooey and melted enough for dunking. Arrange crackers, vegetable crudités, and corn chips to dunk.

Strawberry Fields Forever

I simply adore strawberries. I'm hardly alone. Nutritionist Nancy Farrell, R.D., a spokesperson for the Academy of Nutrition and Dietetics, gets strawberry love. Here is her take on the often-ignored super strawberry.

"Like blueberries, strawberries are versatile. We can place them on top of hot or cold cereal, yogurt or on pancakes. We can blend them in smoothies or add them to a variety of salads. I stress the importance of fiber in strawberries as well. They are fun and easy to eat. Easily transportable in packing a picnic lunch at the park or beach.

"Personally, every year I visit local farms and pick my own strawberries. It is a tradition I do with friends and family. The end result is, of course, strawberry shortcake but the real reason is the homemade strawberry jam I make in large quantities and give as gifts to loved ones. Every spring I get inquiries asking if I am sending more strawberry jam this year."

AVOCADO, THE SUPER BERRY

Surprise. Avocado is not a vegetable; it is a berry and a superfood. This high-fat fruit is loaded with monounsaturated fat, which is the good stuff that improves the "good" cholesterol called high-density lipoprotein (HDL), which protects arteries.

High in calories (258 calories per half an avocado), they are rich in potassium and low in sodium. Avocados do contain a whopping fat count at 27 grams in half of a fruit, but if eaten in moderation the fatty food does have superfood qualities.

Author Fred Pescatore, M.D., M.P.H., based in New York, told me avocado is his favorite superfood. "This is an amazing health food as it provides the healthiest fats," he says, "along with macadamia nuts, olives, and almonds."

His words took me back to my *Woman's World* diet-nutrition columnist days, when I wrote an eye-opening cover story on forward-thinking Barry Sears's high protein diet. It was edgy to hear a doctor dish on tasty high-fat, high-protein foods when low-fat and fat-free foods were "in," so the article likely rocked the dieters' world, as it did mine.

As a kid, I didn't really like the green, mushy avocado slices my mom put into salads. Later, in my twenties, I used a big, rough seed to grow a plant. Then, I learned to make chunky salsa. And that's when I fell in love with the avocado. One hot afternoon, I didn't have much money as a graduate student but I had time on my side during the summer break. I was living in the La Honda mountains (on a route to Santa Cruz, California), and I purchased tomatoes, a fresh onion, and tortillas and used the avocados gifted to me. I peeled the green fruits, chopped them up, and put them into a bowl. I added chopped tomatoes, finely chopped onion, pepper, and salt. Into the fridge it went. I cut and fried tortilla strips in corn oil, and drained them. It was a decadent snack I served to friends later that night. And ever since then the avocado has been loved by me in guacamole, salsa, and some superfood salads.

Super Immune-Boosting Avocado, Strawberry, and Grilled Chicken Salad

This recipe was created by Gemma Sanita Sciabica, my forward-thinking mentor and friend of more than a decade. She used superfoods in both the twentieth and twenty-first centuries. It wasn't until a trip to the Pacific Northwest a few years ago that I noticed sweet and savory salads that are full of deliciousness and superfoods. There's nothing to not like about this California-inspired salad; many of the ingredients come from the Golden State.

For the salad

2 skinless, boneless grilled
   chicken breasts, cut
   into bite-size pieces
½ pound strawberries,
   quartered or sliced
1 or 2 avocados, diced
1 cup blueberries,
   blackberries,
   and/or raspberries

1 kiwi, sliced
1 mango or papaya, diced
1 cup jicama, shredded or
   shaved

For the dressing

¼ cup tangerine or
   orange juice
⅓ cup extra-virgin olive oil
   (Sciabica's or Marsala
   extra-virgin olive oil)
Sea salt and white pepper,
   to taste

¼ cup balsamic vinegar or
   lemon juice
1 cup raspberries
⅓ cup pistachios,
   chopped small
1 4-ounce log goat cheese
   (chèvre)

> Place salad ingredients (except pistachios and cheese) in a large, shallow serving bowl. Set aside. In a blender, combine dressing ingredients, blend until smooth. Drizzle salad with dressing, toss gently. Roll cheese in pistachios, slice. Arrange slices over top of salad.
>
> (Courtesy: Gemma Sanita Sciabica, from *Cooking with California Olive Oil: Recipes from the Heart for the Heart*)

In the next chapter, I'll show you how cheese—yes, cheese, the real artisanal stuff (not fat-free knock-offs)—is not a "bad" food. Cheese, enjoyed in moderation, is the "new" superfood on the block. There are a lot of reasons why I love cheese, and it may be one of your favorite superfoods, too. Take a look at the cheese chapter to see my sobering findings, and you, like me, can discover how to lose the guilt, indulge in your favorite varieties (in moderation), and reap the amazing benefits, which may surprise you.

SUPER-IOR SUPERFOODS FOR THOUGHT

✓ Berries may help lower the risk of developing cancers, lower levels of bad cholesterol, boost immunity, and much more.

✓ Like apples and other superfruits, berries and their healing powers are acknowledged around the world as healing medicines.

✓ Berries, not unlike apples, contain a host of antioxidants that make them functional foods that you are advised to incorporate into your daily diet for good health.

✓ Also, berries are plentiful in dietary fiber and essential nutrients like potassium and contain no fat or sodium, all of which make them super nutritious.

✓ You can enjoy berries year-round in a variety of ways—in fresh, frozen, and dried forms.

Cheese

*How can you govern a country which has 246
varieties of cheese?*
—CHARLES DE GAULLE

Superfruits like berries (all kinds) played a big role in my wonder years, but other food groups—like dairy—were considered super to me as a kid, too. Enter cheese. On Saturday nights my parents would often go out and let a babysitter make an easy dinner. Sometimes, we'd get a Swanson chicken TV dinner or hamburgers and fries. But one night she cooked, sort of. I suppose it was her way to help make my brother and me happy rather than resentful, being left home alone while my parents enjoyed a dinner and movie.

The hip teen (who wore voguish clothes and let us watch *The Twilight Zone*) constructed a double-decker fifties-style grilled cheese sandwich and called it a "toastie." She used Wonder Bread (soft, white, bland cookie-cutter slices, wrapped in a white cellophane wrapper decorated with blue, red, and yellow balls) and processed American cheese slices. In a skillet, the sandwiches were cooked with oleomargarine. The sizzling, crispy brown sandwiches were cut into triangles and served on a plate next to a bowl of Campbell's vegetable soup. I remember the tantalizing crunch of the first bite and can still see the cheesy goo. While it wasn't a twenty-first-century *The Devil Wears Prada* gourmet grilled cheese sandwich dished up by the cute student chef Adrian Grenier, who used eight-dollar Jarlsberg cheese, it *was* a cheese sandwich to love.

THE HISTORY OF CHEESE

Cheese can be upgraded into superfood status by using the right kind and right amount and pairing it with whole-grain bread, leafy greens, and tomatoes. Grilled cheese sandwiches were common kid food in the early twentieth century, and they were budget friendly during the Great Depression. But cheese has a long history.

The making of cheese dates back to four thousand years ago, say food historians. And back to the present day, gourmet grilled cheese sandwiches (made with goat cheese or a mix of cheeses) are often on the menus in popular dives and restaurants around the world.

An Accidental Cheese Discovery

As the legend goes, the art of making cheese was discovered accidentally by an Arabian merchant who put milk into a pouch made from a sheep's stomach as he went on a trek through the desert. This method curdles milk because it reacts with the heat of the sun to make cheese. In the night the traveler was pleasantly surprised that the whey satisfied his thirst, and the cheese (or curd) had a super flavor that appeased his hunger.[1]

SUPER NUTRIENTS

"Cheese is a 'good' food!" I find myself saying to women and men who want to "slim down, healthy up." Cheese is one of my favorite superfoods. Images of the *French Kiss* film heroine (played by Meg Ryan) come to mind, when she is thrilled by the array of cheeses in France. But some nutritionists I interviewed do not believe cheese—any kind—deserves to be included on a healthiest-foods list, let alone tagged a superfood, because of its high fat and high sodium content.

Sure, if you look at the nutrition label of your favorite cheese you may think twice before incorporating it into your diet. But wait, take a look at the nutrition label closer! An ounce (that is a small amount!) of cheddar cheese contains about 110 calories and 9 grams of fat, and most cheeses contain about 20-plus milligrams of cholesterol (less than 10 percent of your daily allowance). Soft cheeses, like goat and ricotta cheeses, often are lower in fat. I am thrilled to differ because medical researchers conclude there is no evidence that shows eating cheese causes heart disease.[2]

In fact, cheese makes the grade in the Oldways Mediterranean Diet Pyramid, and it gets credit by medical researchers for actually lowering the risk of developing heart disease. Cheese in modest amounts provides heart-healthy benefits and also gives much more to its loyal followers around the globe—not just those in France and Italy. Choose natural cheese for the best flavor and superfood nutrients. But there's more!

HEALTH BENEFITS OF CHEESE

Cheese is a super source of calcium, which is good for calming your nervous system and for your teeth and bones. Past medical research shows that people who get an adequate amount of calcium by eating a moderate amount of dairy, which includes cheese, may be likely to keep their blood pressure numbers in check—lowering their risk of heart disease and stroke.

Not only can cheese be heart-healthy, it may even do more for your health. One study by researchers at the University of South Korea and published in the journal *Current Microbiology* revealed not only the nutritional bonanza of cheese but also its probiotic powers, thanks to *Propionibacterium freudenreichii*, which is key to enhancing the immune system and boosting longevity.[3]

So, cheese people around the globe can give a collective sigh of relief, eat their cheese, and enjoy it, too! Cheddar, feta, Gouda, Swiss, and hundreds of other cheeses have gotten a bad rap because of their saturated fat content, but in moderation, real cheese boasts a myriad of nutritional and health benefits that you may not know about, and it's time to listen up and crunch some in-the-know cheese numbers.

Cheese Is an Ignored Superfood

The choices of superfoods are debated, but it didn't take long for me to discover the super health perks of cheese (different types) cited by past and present diet wizards. Nutritionist Nancy Farrell, R.D., for one, not only likes strawberries, but she also agrees that there are benefits of some types of cheese, too.

Lately my favorite cheese is Stilton cheese with apricots. A nice addition to an adult cheese, vegetables, and a cracker platter served with red wine. Many people don't care for Swiss cheese, but I have fond memories of eating it with my father. Actually, 80 percent of our food choices are psychological and based on childhood remembrances. So it is important to get our children up for success with foods and eating.

We are a global world and we should encourage our children to continue to try new foods all the time as most assuredly they will be traveling. Teaching our kids how to cook and to appreciate different tasting foods lasts a lifetime.

Back to Swiss cheese . . . Hard cheeses, like Swiss, Provolone, Parmesan, Cheddar, are more easily digested for those who are lactose intolerant.

In my decades of experience, people either love or hate cottage cheese. Yet cottage cheese is frequently seen in weight loss meal plans. And what's up with ricotta cheese? Can you interchange the two? It depends on your health and food product needs. Cottage cheese is made from curds and ricotta is made from whey protein. Reduced-fat ricotta has more calories and fat per serving, but it doesn't have the lumps so prominent (and deemed unpleasant by many) in cottage cheese. Keep in mind, cottage cheese has a higher liquid content than ricotta, so the recipe (think cheesecake, dips, lasagna) really dictates which is best to use.

Cheese Numbers Good to Know

It's good to be in the know about taste and texture in cheese, but just as important is noting the fat and sodium content in your picks for uses from simple snacking to serious cooking and delicious baking.

Here is a quick rundown of some of the good stuff—including protein and calcium—in various cheeses. Keep in mind, there are other nutritional and health benefits of cheese. (See the chapters on weight loss, aging, home cures, and recipes.) Yes, you can eat your favorite cheese and enjoy it, too, without the guilt, as people in France do.

Cheese (*1 ounce unless specified*)	Calories (*grams*)	Fat (*grams*)	Protein (*grams*)	Sodium (*mgms*)	Calcium (*mgms*)
Blue Cheese	6	110	6	395	149
Cheddar	114	9.5	7	176	204
Cottage Cheese, 1% fat (1 cup)	113	2.5	28	917	137
Goat	76	6	5	232	39.5
Parmesan, grated	111	8.5	12	528	390
Swiss	106	8	8	73	272

(Source: Manufacturers' Labels)

There are so many varieties of cheese to choose from, but I must say some do not make the grade with me—super or not. On a trip to Vancouver, British Columbia, I took the bus from Seattle versus the train to change things up a bit with a scenic route. It was picturesque, but after a few hours I suffered a bout of motion sickness. At the U.S.–Canada border there is a small store. I was greeted with chocolate and cookies like a sequel of the film *The Twilight Zone*, segment two.

By the time I arrived at the hotel, all I could think of was to get something to eat. Before checking in I sat down at the café and ordered a grilled cheese sandwich on whole wheat and chamomile tea. I nibbled on strange crackers while waiting for my comfort food. The presentation of the sandwich was perfect—until I took a bite. "What is in this cheese?" I asked the waitress because something was off. "It's smoked goat cheese." I assumed it would be mild cheddar or Monterey Jack. Unhappy and queasy, I sipped tea and vowed never to eat that type of cheese, while out of the country or even back home in California.

Since that upset tummy episode passed, I've eaten a wide variety of cheese types, including goat cheese—minus the smoked variety.

At home, I decided to give regular goat cheese another try for fig appetizers, a superfood treat wherever you are. Slicing fresh figs in half, spreading the tops with soft goat cheese, topping with nuts (chopped hazelnuts or almonds), and drizzling with raw honey makes an afternoon delight, and for me, it makes up for the Canadian afternoon of a sandwich nondelight.

The wide world of cheese is one to explore. Not only will you get a plethora of vitamins and minerals from a delicious and versatile superfood, but by pairing different types of cheese with other superfoods, like in a salad, you also will enter Superfoodland.

Super Healing Tomato and Mozzarella Salad

6 to 8 Belgian endive, Boston lettuce, or radicchio leaves
4 tomatoes, sliced
4 hard-boiled eggs
1 onion, sliced into thin rings
2 avocados, sliced into rings

2 cups olives, sliced
8 thin slices mozzarella
¼ cup lime or lemon juice
⅓ cup olive oil (Marsala olive fruit oil)
Salt, pepper, and paprika, to taste
½ cup fresh basil, chopped

Line large platter with lettuce leaves. Arrange tomatoes, eggs, onions, avocados, olives, and mozzarella slices overlapping on lettuce in serving platter. Save some olives for garnish. In small bowl, whisk together juice, oil, salt, pepper, and paprika. Spoon juice and oil mixture evenly over salad, sprinkle with basil. Garnish with olives.

Makes 6–8 servings.
(Courtesy: Gemma Sanita Sciabica, from *Cooking with Olive Oil: Treasured Family Recipes*)

If you love cheese, you may not like what's up next—green super-foods. Keep an open mind as I reintroduce crucifers (broccoli, cauli-flower, and kale) that I, and maybe you, have turned your nose up to as a kid or a grown-up. Those past leafy greens (toss the iceberg lettuce you fed to the pet bird or lizard) may bore you, but these updated veg-etables are my superfood companions and have been for decades. Turn the pages ahead to find out exactly why these veggies made it to my fa-vorite superfoods list and, I hope, will make it into your diet regime, one way or another.

SUPER-IOR HEALING SUPERFOODS FOR THOUGHT

✓ Cheese may help you lower the risk of developing cancers, reduce levels of bad cholesterol, boost immunity, and much more.
✓ Each kind of cheese is acknowledged by medical researchers as a healing food that has a variety of healing powers.
✓ Cheese contains a lot of vitamins and minerals and it can be paired with other superfoods, making it a wholesome, versatile superfood.
✓ But you should eat less cheese rather than more to get the super healing benefits.

Crucifers (and Leafy Greens)

> *Training is everything. The peach was once a*
> *bitter almond; cauliflower is nothing but cabbage*
> *with a college education.*
> —MARK TWAIN, *Pudd'nhead Wilson*

Before traveling as an adult throughout the decades, vegetables did play a role (thanks to their pound-paring powers) in my diet during my self-conscious teenage years. Thanks to acne and baby fat, I was comforted by cookies to cope with peer-pressure challenges. While a grilled cheese would win over veggies, I did eat the green stuff to fight the hormones. In the mid-twentieth century, canned green beans and frozen green peas were the green vegetables I remember pushing to the side of the plate in dishes. But we also were no strangers to fresh greens since we did live in the Valley of Heart's Delight, which was chock-full of California's best lettuce, artichokes, and broccoli—all somewhat more suitable to a kid's palate.

One birthday party in particular stands out in my stash of super-food memories as a tween. On a Saturday afternoon, I sat down to a large vintage table in the rustic dining room of my friend's home. Her mother was more frugal and down-to-earth than mine was. When the food was brought out to the table I was pleasantly surprised. A large tuna salad filled with a variety of lettuces and tomatoes and a home-made thousand island made it to my plate. Homemade bread and but-ter were also part of the luncheon. "This was the best salad I've ever eaten!" I exclaimed to my mom that night, asking if she would make a salad for *my* birthday party in the fall.

My mother followed up with an amazing and sophisticated kid-friendly Cobb salad (with the magical flair of Dr. Seuss's *Green Eggs and Ham*). The super salad included a mix of leafy greens, avocado slices, chicken, eggs, and Jack cheese—all drizzled with a perfect ranch dressing. And that was the day when I fell in love with greens. A buffet-style lunch with salad, cornbread, and a chocolate birthday cake was served on the picnic table. Despite my dad being grumpy about the lawn being trampled by thirty kids, it was a superfoods day.

These days, I often choose a grown-up plate of greens at a restau-rant; a house salad, one with baby greens, pear, blue cheese, pecans, cranberries, and a vinaigrette, will suffice in a heartbeat. Not to ignore a repurposed chef's salad (with different cheeses as add-ons and cru-ciferous vegetables for the health of it) for the new century and new superfoods.

THE HISTORY OF CRUCIFERS

Cruciferous vegetables (*Brassica oleracea*), including my superfood choices—broccoli, cauliflower, and kale—belong to the cabbage fam-ily. They are nothing new; in fact, these superveggies can be traced back centuries. Around the first century A.D., cabbage was introduced to the world. Around the fifth century B.C., kale was discovered. By the fifteenth century A.D., cauliflower was being eaten in Europe, followed by broccoli in Italy a century later.

While crucifers and leafy greens have been around for centuries, people of all ages didn't always love these veggies, crucifers being on the bottom of the list or blacklisted. But due to their superfood health benefits, the superfoods ongoing trend, and people's creativity in cooking and serving vegetable dishes, it's time to give these gems an-other chance to be included in your favorite superfoods choices.

SUPER NUTRIENTS

Broccoli: Medical researchers show that this anticancer vegetable deserves its credit for a variety of its super nutrients. This dark-green vegetable is plentiful in the antioxidant carotene and the mineral calcium, it is very low in fat, plus it contains dietary fiber, too—all good things for fighting cancer and heart disease.

Cauliflower: This white crucifer takes a while to warm up to. (When I was a kid, I'd give it to the dog under the table.) But as a diet-conscious woman, I began to like the white stuff because it was low in calories, fat, and sodium. One cup of cauliflower contains potassium and fiber to help fill you up not out. Once your palate matures and/or health is on your brain, you may want to prepare it in tasty ways (often with broccoli) to get all of the super nutrition and health perks.

Kale: Enter another crucifer that I did not try until recently. First, I purchased a large package of the solo stuff (it was organic) and brought it home. It looked big, curly, and a bit strange. I went back to the supermarket and grabbed a bag of mixed greens; spinach and kale were part of the deal. It was like at first bite; nowadays it is love. I adore the blend of spinach and kale for the different flavors and textures. Both greens are always in my vegetable bin and enjoyed every week. (My meat-and-potatoes sibling who used to eat iceberg lettuce—a dietary death sentence for an iguana because it lacks nutrients—now eats kale, too!)

Kale has plentiful carotenes (lutein and zeaxanthin)—those heart-healthy antioxidants I mentioned in Chapter 1. Also, not only does kale contain heart-healthy minerals like calcium and potassium (those are super for keeping our blood pressure in check), but that's not where it stops. Kale also contain folate, the B vitamin that helps lower levels of homocysteine, the blood factor that can wreak havoc on our arteries. Not to forget, kale also boasts vitamin C, another heart-healthy antioxidant. While kale is a powerhouse of nutrients, I truly love the taste and texture of it. But there's more . . .

This antioxidant-rich superfood rates number one on that popular oxygen radical absorbance capacity (ORAC) chart. In the vegetable category, kale ranks at 1,770 (above spinach at 1,200). So, since they're both good for you, why not mix them together and get the best of nutrients, texture, and flavor?

HEALTH BENEFITS OF CRUCIFERS

The American Cancer Society, medical researchers, *and* doctors (including an oncologist I interviewed for *Woman's World* magazine for an article on breast cancer) will tell you why the vegetables of the cabbage family, broccoli and cauliflower included, are touted as top cancer fighters. Credit is given to the fiber and antioxidants, called indoles, found in these two vegetables, which can be enjoyed raw and dipped in yogurt for snacks, and used in salads, casseroles, soups, side dishes, and stir-frys.

My mom used to trickle melted cheddar cheese on cauliflower, which I *would* eat. Nowadays, a popular cauliflower trend is to cook it up like mashed potatoes. Try mashing cooked cauliflower with a bit of fresh lemon, sea salt, ground pepper, and chives. Add a small amount of real butter, and an anticauliflower individual may become a crucifer convert for its health perks and flavor.

Also, both cauliflower and broccoli contain folate, which may help lower your risk of developing heart disease. Past research has shown that people with more folate in their diet can lose weight more easily, and this, in turn, could make crucifers more heart-healthy because by losing unwanted pounds you can help keep your blood pressure numbers in check. While crucifers can be an acquired taste (I often include both broccoli and cauliflower in salads), leafy greens (a dieter's dream food) deserve a place in favorite superfoods, too.

THE HISTORY OF LEAFY GREENS

It is believed that the Greeks and Romans, way back in time, enjoyed dishes with raw vegetables dressed with herbs, oil, and vinegar—more superfoods. Not to ignore the medicinal practitioners, too, such as Hippocrates and Galen, who believed that raw veggies easily slipped through the digestive system and did not create obstructions. And this finding may be the genesis of leafy greens served as the popular dinner salad before the entrée in a meal, per doctors' orders for health's sake.[1]

Back in the fifties and sixties, iceberg lettuce (the light green vegetable) was sold at supermarkets in lettuce heads (big balls) to be washed and chopped, used as a topping with a sliced tomato on hamburgers at drive-thru fast-food chains, and even as the main lettuce during the salad hoopla in the seventies—a health era when sprouts and seeds were "in" at health food stores and as hippies' favorite foods during the macrobiotic fad.

SUPER NUTRIENTS

Nowadays, while iceberg lettuce may be part of a salad mix or served at an old-fashioned sandwich shop, it is not the super salad green of choice. Dark-green leafy greens, though, such as spinach, are the super vegetables of the twenty-first century and are gaining popularity, thanks to their super nutritional value and taste when paired with other super greens for more flavor and texture. Leafy greens all are low in calories and fat. But the darker ones contain vitamins and minerals that are better for you. They are a mere 12 calories per one cup (raw) and are full of vitamin A, vitamin C, and fiber, and are low in fat and rich in iron. What else could a dieter or salad lover crave, right?

HEALTH BENEFITS OF LEAFY GREENS

Raw baby spinach has been a staple in my diet for many years. It's been my go-to salad base at home and when I'm on the road, at cafes and restaurants. Not to leave out the fact that paired with cheese (feta, Swiss or cheddar), sunflower seeds, Roma tomatoes, and a vinaigrette, it's heaven and healthy. It's a no brainer that it's heart-healthy because it's low in fat and dietary fiber, which can help lower cholesterol levels. But it's brain food, too!

Eating one serving per day of green leafy vegetables may help slow cognitive decline and keep your mind sharper. Researchers doing a study published in the journal *Neurology* gave a questionnaire to 960 people (ages 58–99) in a memory and aging project for almost five years. The findings: Eating greens showed a slower decline in brain function. The conclusion: The researchers give health credit to the nutrients, including vitamin K, lutein, B-carotene, folate, and others.[2]

Mainstream consumers know both spinach and crucifers are on the popular superfoods list. But, according to nutritionist Robin

Foroutan, R.D., spokesperson for the Academy of Nutrition and Dietetics, there is no need to exclude other salad greens (such as chard, parsley, and watercress) to make a super salad bowl. This way, you're getting more super nutrients, flavor, and texture in your salads. Foroutan explains that in the Persian culture, meals are served with a platter full of *sabzi*, meaning greens. Sabzi platters include salad greens and basil, mint, and radishes with their green tops attached— and sometimes, feta cheese—for people to enjoy with their meal. "The freshness and intense flavors of the herbs," she explains, "cleanse the palate" and go well with quality protein sources like fish. And if eating salads bore you, it's time to go to green drinks.

Super Health-Boosting Hidden Greens Smoothie

I've watched Hallmark Channel films where health-minded characters are portrayed drinking dark-green smoothies and observers are not eager to join in and swallow the blended-iguana look-alike beverage. One woman claimed her green lizard-colored drink would clean her chakras (look it up in a new age dictionary). This Hidden Greens Smoothie had me at the super-foods mix of crucifers and superfruits—not just greens like kale. But I like to take it slow, so I used ¼ cup kale salad mix (containing cabbage) for a lighter-green-colored smoothie.

8 ounces purified water or cran-water
1 scoop powdered vanilla whey or Body Protein (Fat Flush)
1 scoop powdered probiotic
½ cup kale

½ cup cauliflower
½ cup mixed berries
5 frozen cherries, pitted
Ice cubes (optional)
1 tablespoon coconut oil
1 tablespoon chia seeds
Zest of 1 lemon

Combine water, whey, probiotic, vegetables, fruits, and ice in a blender until smooth. Add the coconut oil, chia seeds, and lemon zest. Blend until all ingredients are incorporated.

Makes 1 serving.
(Courtesy: Ann Louise Gittleman, Ph.D., C.N.S.)

Getting your greens on can be exciting, especially when you pair a variety with other superfoods—including the egg! Up next, I'll show you how eggs—the "new" comeback healing food—get a thumbs-up. Take a look at the incredible egg; open your eyes to this superfood that can be put to work for both your body and mind (and it's good for beautifying treatments, as shown in Chapter 26!).

SUPER-IOR HEALING SUPERFOODS FOR THOUGHT

✓ Cruciferous vegetables may help lower the risk of developing cancers, reduce levels of bad cholesterol, boost immunity, and much more.

✓ Leafy greens are eaten around the world and acknowledged as healing medicines.

✓ Crucifers mixed with greens can double their healing powers in a variety of ways—thanks to their antioxidants and other amazing properties.

✓ Incorporating a variety of greens in your diet will help to add more nutrients to your food, and don't forget your enjoyment of their super flavors, different textures, and versatile uses.

✓ Crucifers and leafy greens aren't just for salads: Think outside of the salad bowl and use them for soups, smoothies, and casseroles, and with main dishes such as fish and pasta.

CHAPTER
7

Eggs

*The bird fights his way out of the egg. The egg is
the world.*
—HERMAN HESSE, *Demian*

Salads and crucifers go together like salt and pepper, but eggs, like the
raw ones in a Caesar salad, were not my favorite egg treat in my childhood. It was the baked egg custard event, though, that had me at the
first crack of the egg. In eighth grade, my home economics class assigned us to make an easy dessert. I chose custard because I knew it
was "fail-proof." All the ingredients were in the kitchen: whole milk,
eggs, sugar, vanilla, and nutmeg. Using just the egg yolks (separating
eggs was a challenge), warming the liquid on the stovetop, and pour-
ing the light-yellow stuff into glass ramekins was fun. When my
mother asked me what I was doing, I answered, "Homework. I'm making egg custard." She exhaled. In retrospect, she likely knew this simple egg recipe wouldn't leave her kitchen looking like a scene from the
film *Twister*, complete with flying cows. The end result: The egg custard would be edible.

As I grew up, my egg love blossomed to eating and liking dishes like
quiche lorraine and egg-white frittata, and scrambling two vegetarian

cage-free eggs paired with shredded cheese, tomatoes, and fresh herbs and spices is my cup of tea, sweet and simple on Sunday mornings.

THE HISTORY OF EGGS

As food historians will tell you, bird eggs—all kinds, including from the chicken—have been used as food since prehistoric times. The chicken was most likely used for its eggs before 7500 B.C. Later, the egg was brought to Sumer, Egypt, and then Greece by 1500 B.C.[1]

In ancient Rome, eggs were used in many ways, and meals often began with an egg course. Not only have eggs been eaten since caveman days, but they also are still enjoyed today in many ways for their convenience and wide variety of nutritional merits.[2]

SUPER NUTRIENTS

Nutritionists will tell you the egg has gotten a bad rap because of its high cholesterol, but as nutritionist Robin Foroutan, R.D., points out, "In moderation this versatile superfood is one that deserves a place in a superfood repertoire." And nutritious eggs—the real food from a real chicken—are applauded today in many diets for good reason.

Chicken eggs (cage-free eggs are recommended by health experts for both the chicken and human!) provide 155 calories and 12 grams of protein. Eggs contain vitamin B_{12} and vitamin D.

Egg yolk is also high in vitamins A and E. Egg white contain 20 percent of the egg's calories, and it has no fat. I recall that when I was a teen on the stay-skinny track to mimic the picture-perfect size-two magazine models, I ate more rather than less egg whites and tossed the yolks. This smart feat didn't make my budget-smart mom smile. And in my thirties, a body builder insisted I eat egg whites like he did to help bulk up my arms while working out with free weights. (I give credit to the extra protein, but the workouts also helped when I was on a mission to get Linda Hamilton arms, as seen in *Terminator* films.) But times change, and the reputation of egg yolks has changed for the twenty-first century.

HEALTH BENEFITS OF EGGS

Research results published in *The Journal of the American Medical Association* revealed the healthful benefits of the touted incredible egg. In two studies that included almost forty thousand men and more than eighty thousand women, scientists found that eating eggs in moderation (one per day) was not linked to heart disease in healthy people.[3]

What's more, the American Heart Association says if you're healthy, it's all right to eat up to four eggs a week. So the jury is still out on the exact amount of eggs to eat—less is more—but they are certainly worth incorporating in a heart-healthy diet.

Foroutan, like other food experts, understands the new superfood status of eggs, "especially the yolk." She says, "Go for the whole egg as nature intended. The yolks are super high in choline which is great for brain health." She adds that the best way to protect the healthy fats in the yolk is to cook eggs on low heat, which will help protect the "integrity of the fat" and that "poached and hard or soft boiled eggs are healthier cooking methods because they protect the fats from oxidizing during the cooking process."

The egg-savvy food expert shares her favorite way to begin her day is with eggs—the whole egg. She keeps hard-boiled, peeled eggs in the refrigerator so that she can "grab and eat on the go." On late work nights when cooking is another job, she'll simply whip up scrambled eggs and pair them with a super salad bowl complete with avocado and tomato.

Personally, I prefer organic brown eggs (these days I do eat the white and yolk) and 100 percent cage-free ones. As a lacto-vegetarian, I turn to eggs (in moderation) as a source for protein. Egg salad sandwiches paired with greens and hard-boiled eggs in a variety of salads are excellent, and when they are paired with other superfoods, they provide a super variety of nutrients, flavor, and texture. And note, cooking eggs lowers the risk of bacteria problems; this is why I stay clear of adding raw eggs in dishes, but baked in recipes they are my favorite.

Super Stimulating Vegetable Cheesy Quiche

❖ ❖ ❖

As a kid, my mom served quiche. I didn't touch it. My ten-year-old palate was ready for hard-boiled Easter eggs, not a fancy European gooey yellow pie. Decades later, not only did the sense of belonging to French and English culture come to me (via my visits to Quebec and British Columbia), but quiche also grew to be one of my favorite superfood dishes for breakfast, brunch, dinner, and even a late-night snack. This recipe is European-inspired, with my mother's taste for sophisticated cuisine.

1 tablespoon olive oil

1 tablespoon European-style butter

4 tablespoons red onion, chopped

1¼ cups broccoli and cauliflower florets, chopped

1 tablespoon fresh basil, chopped

3 organic eggs, lightly beaten

1½ cups organic half-and-half

Black pepper and sea salt, to taste

1 (9-inch) premium store-bought refrigerated piecrust

½ cup premium organic mozzarella, shredded

½ cup premium organic Monterey Jack, shredded

2 heirloom or Roma tomatoes, sliced

¼ cup pine nuts

In a skillet, melt olive oil and butter. Stir-fry onion and vegetables. Add basil. Set aside. In a mixing bowl, combine eggs and half-and-half. Add pepper and salt. Bake piecrust covered in foil 15 minutes in 400-degree F oven. (This keeps it flaky.) Chill in freezer about 15 minutes. Line piecrust bottom with cheese. Stir lightly so that it's even. Add eggs. Bake at 350 degrees F, 40–45 minutes, or until eggs are firm and crust is a light golden brown. Do not overbake. Cool at least 30 minutes. You can serve warm or chilled. Garnish with tomatoes and nuts.

This quiche works cold for breakfast (the ingredients are more flavorful, cutting it is easy, and perfect slices are the result). Or warm it up for brunch or dinner so the cheese melts and pleases the palate. Serve solo or pair with a tossed green salad with a tangy vinaigrette.

Makes 8–10 servings.

Now that you get that eggs have made a revival, in the next chapter, I'll show you how yogurt gets two thumbs-up in studies by nutritionists, from consumers—and from me. It's the thick, creamy texture that appeases my taste buds—making it a superior superfood to eat. While Greek yogurt has some must-dos to keep it healthy, it can be a superfood.

SUPER-IOR HEALING SUPERFOODS FOR THOUGHT

✓ The versatile egg, with its array of good-for-you nutrients, may help lower the risk of developing cancers, reduce levels of bad cholesterol, boost immunity, and much more.

✓ Eggs, especially organic ones from free-range, antibiotic- and preservative-free chickens, have healing powers and are acknowledged around the world as healing medicines.

✓ Eggs help boost brainpower thanks to their protein and fatty acids.

✓ The ancient egg, with its vitamins and minerals, is here to stay in the twenty-first century, and it's part of the heart-healthy diet.

CHAPTER

8

Greek Yogurt (and Gelato)

A human can be healthy without killing animals
for food.
—LEO NIKOLAEVICH TOLSTOY

Protein-rich eggs and yogurt found their way into my diet as a shy teenager who wanted to be lean with long, straight hair—not curly locks. Yogurt was a new health food to me, with the promise of superpowers to get me skinny like the supermodels. In the sixties, it was the fad to wear miniskirts and two-piece bathing suits. In high school, I loved wearing eye-catching outfits, but I needed to drop unwanted pounds by replacing cookies and chips. One day I made the decision to give yogurt (a food made by the fermentation of milk) a try like the diet gurus. I tried the low-fat type with fruit on the bottom. At first, it was like tasting black tea or coffee (two more superfoods touted to help burn fat), and it was not tasty to my unsophisticated palate. It was an acquired taste, but after a few weeks I acquired it because I was on track to a svelte body.

An unforgettable event still makes me smile. My older sister let me wear her green-and-yellow polka-dot miniskirt, complete with bloomers. It was fun drawing attention—until I was sent to the principal's office. The middle-aged woman with power took me into a room with a full-length mirror. She flaunted a long, white measuring tape and measured the length of my skirt to my knee. "Your bloomers are seven inches above the knees. It is not acceptable attire." I darted, "I eat yucky yogurt so I can wear outfits like this!" The petty woman clad in an unflattering dark-colored dress said, "Go home and change your clothes." As I opened the door, the stout but pretty authority figure sheepishly asked, "Yogurt? So, what brand do you eat? I need to lose twenty pounds."

Then and now, I give credit to yogurt, a slimming superfood for all ages. I don't wear miniskirts these days, but I fit into size four skinny jeans (no muffin top, except after a bakefest during the winter holidays). However, my choice of types of yogurt has changed.

During the nineties, when I wrote diet articles, the nutritionists I teamed with preferred to include fat-free yogurt. Ugh! We were going through a fat-free craze (from diet drinks to cheese). The fat-free food—including low-fat yogurt—tasted bland, not delectable like food with fat. But it wasn't until the twenty-first century that I met Greek yogurt and "fell in like" for a variety of reasons, and I'll explain how it made the cut on my 20 Superfoods list.

THE HISTORY OF GREEK YOGURT

The consensus is that historical reports about the roots of Greek yogurt go back to the Neolithic people of Central Asia in 6000 B.C. Also, my personal history is linked to a yogurt factory in New York known as Dannon, which is the first brand of yogurt I saw in the supermarket and tasted in the United States. The popularity of yogurt grew in the 1950s and 1960s, but it first made its mark at health food stores. In twenty-first-century supermarkets, there are an array of brands and types of yogurt, including low-fat and fat-free varieties. But it's Greek yogurt that is gaining popularity—and for good reason.

The Legend of Greek Yogurt

Food historians will tell you that Greek yogurt goes way, way back in time to Bulgaria. It got some recognition by the Thracians, a group of tribes that ruled the Balkans during the Roman era. Ancient warriors carried sheep's milk in lambskins around their bodies. This, in result, helped warm up the temperature to ferment the milk into yogurt. And so the thick, creamy, good-for-you Greek yogurt became more popular. And today, some Bulgarians will credit their longevity to the wondrous dairy foodstuff.

NUTRIENTS IN GREEK YOGURT

Greek yogurt, unlike regular, low-fat, and fat-free types, is made from strained whole milk, which reduces it of liquid whey, lactose, and sugar. However, the Greek variety is made from milk that has been mixed with cream to add fat. A one-cup serving of plain Greek yogurt (depending on the brand) is an excellent source of calcium.

With twice the protein and half the sugar of low-fat or fat-free sweetened yogurts, plain Greek yogurt is more of a superfood. It has more protein and more calcium, not to negate the thick, creamy texture and taste. The best brands will contain no artificial flavors. What's more, Greek yogurt and the demand for it have soared in both the United States and Canada. I recall back in the sixties, Graham Kerr, the charming chef in *The Galloping Gourmet* TV program, was a strained yogurt fan.

HEALTH BENEFITS OF YOGURT

Like cheese, Greek yogurt and regular yogurt are superfoods—and taste great drizzled with raw honey or mixed with fresh fruit. In moderation, this dairy staple is touted for its heart-healthy powers, bone-boosting merits, and immunity-enhancing perks thanks to its probiotics. Plain Greek yogurt is also rich in the mineral potassium. Both calcium and potassium may help you keep your blood pressure and cholesterol numbers in check.[1]

Remember, you want to consume yogurt that has live cultures, which can help the immune system to aid digestive woes. When purchasing Greek yogurt, look at the seal of your container. The acronym LAC (Live and Active Culture) will let you know that your choice of

Greek Yogurt, Plain (unsweetened, whole milk)

Nutrition Facts:
Serving Size: 1 8-ounce cup (21 g)
Amount per Serving:
Calories: 220
Protein: 9.0 g
Saturated Fat: 9.0 mg
Trans Fat: 0 g
Cholesterol: 50 mg
Sodium: 150 mg
Calcium: 100 g. 35% Daily Value
Vitamin A: 10% Daily Value
Phosphorous: 30% Daily Value
Potassium: 460 mg
Sugars: 15 g
(*Source:* Excerpt from Nutrient Data Laboratory, ARS, USDA; National Nutrient Database 28)

yogurt is blessed with the good stuff, much like the great "mother" in apple cider vinegar.

Flavored Greek yogurts are decadent, but there is a not-so-sweet catch. That sweet strawberry or honey Greek yogurt that you may walk a mile for contains a whopping amount of added sugar—more than 20 grams in one cup. (The American Heart Association recommends no more than 36 grams of sugar for men and 20 grams for women per day.)

But you can get your daily dose of Greek yogurt deliciousness and eat it, too, if you choose wisely. That means, pick plain, unsweetened yogurt. Add it to a smoothie or a cup of fresh berries, top a potato, or eat it plain with a bit of raw honey. You'll get used to the plain variety versus the flavored types. It's still a super tasting superfood, and its creamy, thick texture isn't going anywhere. If you're a fan of Greek yogurt, gelato will be another super delight.

Greek yogurt brands are easy to find in your local supermarket, supercenters, health food stores, and, of course, you can make it yourself. In my early twenties, I traveled with a friend to the suburbs of Chicago. When his mom opened the refrigerator I couldn't help but notice a bowl with a cloth over it. I asked, "What's that?" The middle-aged woman was making yogurt. Back then I thought it seemed like a lot of work since you could buy it at the store. But she also conserved water, used compost, and made apple butter from the apple tree in the backyard. I got it. It was a time of self-reliance and making your own yogurt for the thrill of it all.

GELATO AND ICE CREAM

Gelato is often called an Italian ice cream, but it is more than that, according to ice cream and frozen dessert proponents who make and sell the delight. The delicious ice cream spin-off is a mixture of milk, cream, and sugar, and is often flavored with fruit and nuts. It may be considered a "new" superfood because when you eat it in moderation you are getting less fat and often more natural ingredients than in ice cream.

. Its roots are derived from ancient Rome and Egypt. Food historians claim it came from snow and ice brought down from mountaintops by locals. In the early twentieth century, the first gelato was developed in the United States.

I recall in the 1980s I tasted my first cup of gelato, chocolate chip, at a quaint ice cream shop in Marin, California. The texture of the dessert was creamy, rich, and decadent. Later on, in the twenty-first century, gelato made its mark in mainstream supermarkets, with plenty of brand-name competition. These days, northern California has many hot spots that offer a variety of superfood ice creams, gelatos, and sorbets in distinctive flavors, including edamame lemon, mascarpone kumquat, Meyer lemon rose, and strawberry balsamic beet.

I've discovered, too, if you turn to making homemade gelato, ice cream, or sorbet by using an ice cream maker, you can end up with a DIY superfood. If you make it yourself, you control the ingredients and can be creative by adding other superfoods! Try olive oil and dark chocolate, chai or matcha powder, or sweet potato and honey. Making these treats can soar to superfood heights and the varieties are limitless.

THE SCOOP ON ICE CREAM

Some research suggests ice cream may be considered a new superfood. Not only is it rich in bone-boosting calcium and protein (good for muscle mass, hair, and teeth), but it has other super nutrients, too. Vanilla ice cream contains choline, a mineral that enhances brain function. This food is low in sodium but high in saturated fat, so portion control is important.[2]

Also, ever notice how both women and men will eat ice cream when they're feeling down after an emotional upset? Well, research shows ice cream may diminish the brain's response to sadness. Scientists at the University of Leuven in Belgium discovered mood-boosting benefits of ice cream, and their findings were published in the *Journal of Clinical Investigation*.[3]

Twelve healthy people allowed to have their brains scanned using an MRI to show the effect of the body on the mind. The volunteers were given a fatty solution through a feeding tube. Then, they listened to a sad or neutral classical music song while viewing images of human facial expressions showing sadness or a neutral expression. The findings were that the fatty solution in ice cream can lower sadness, lessen hunger, and increase mood positivity.

Homemade ice cream is an ideal way to control the ingredients and make it a superfood. Using other superfoods, including ingredients such as berries, chai, dark chocolate, nuts, olive oil, seeds, or matcha powder can make ice cream amazing. I prefer recipes that don't use eggs. Ice cream makers will make this superfood a reality if you choose one that is easy to use and is without glitches.

Another route to take is to choose premium store-bought ice cream—all natural, less sugar, and ingredients you can pronounce. Some popular brands give you superfood ice cream, such as Häagen-

Dazs, for one. It offers a line of five flavors (chocolate, vanilla, strawberry, coffee, and green tea) that contain only five ingredients. Organic and vegan brands are also available to you.

Or do it yourself and choose your favorite brand of ready-made all-natural ice cream, let it soften at room temperature, add superfoods, and put in the freezer to rechill. Fold in fresh berries, nuts, raw honey and mascarpone cheese, natural creamy peanut butter, and dark chocolate chips. You'll have semihomemade superfood ice cream without the time and effort of using an ice cream maker. Using gelato or ice cream instead of yogurt to make it sweet and provide a thick and creamy texture can work, too.

Super Energizing Cherry-Almond Smoothie

❖ ❖ ❖

We always keep the ingredients for this smoothie on hand, and it's incredibly adaptable for pretty much any kind of frozen fruit-and-nut combination you have on hand. Blueberries and pecans? Bananas and walnuts? Apricots and pistachios? Try them all! None will be overwhelmed by the additional maple syrup, and you can increase or decrease the sweetness to your liking.

½ cup vanilla or plain Greek yogurt
½ cup frozen cherries
1 tablespoon maple syrup (Crown Maple, very dark color, strong taste)
1 tablespoon ground almonds or ground flax seeds

2 tablespoons almond milk
½ teaspoon almond extract
½ teaspoon vanilla extract

Blend all the ingredients—yogurt, cherries, syrup, almonds or seeds, milk, and extracts—together in a blender
until smooth. Taste and add more maple syrup for additional sweetness if you'd like, or more almond milk for a
milkier consistency. Pour into a glass and serve.

Makes 1 serving.
(Courtesy: Crown Maple and *The Crown Maple Guide
to Maple Syrup*)

Later on, you'll discover that yogurt is a multipurpose superfood—
not just something you eat!. Meanwhile, let's take a look at lemons—
not the superfood orange. While oranges are a citrus favorite, the
magical lemon is a favorite superfood in my book and is not to be
snubbed.

SUPER-IOR HEALING SUPERFOODS FOR THOUGHT

✓ Greek yogurt, with its powers, is accepted around the world as a
healing medicine.
✓ Yogurt, not unlike other superfoods, heals in a variety of ways—
thanks to its antioxidants, calcium, probiotics, and other amazing
properties.
✓ Greek yogurt has a multitude of uses (even topically), but as a
superfood to eat it is definitely worth trying (if you haven't expanded your yogurt types), and you may be pleasantly surprised
by its delicious thick, creamy texture.
✓ It gets even better when added to smoothies, used with superfruits and vegetables, and cooking and baking with it, too.
✓ Greek yogurt is high in calories, and if flavored high in sugar. For
a healthier yogurt, use a plain Greek variety and add a bit of raw
honey.

Lemons

Under the lemon tart
Who loves to lie with me.
—WILLIAM SHAKESPEARE, *As You Like It*

During my early twenties, it was a seventies phenomenon to eat yogurt and fruit and hitchhike across America. One summer I was stranded in Tennessee, headed to the Florida Keys. Tired from a long day of heat, I caught a ride from a man who resembled a well-groomed country singer. He was aloof to me and my Lhasa Apso/Maltese mix dog, Tiger. When the quiet man stopped the car and requested me to go outside in the dark to check the back tire, my four-legged companion jumped out after me. The man sped off with my worldly possessions: a knapsack, sleeping bag, and purse with doggie treats. Bam! There I stood in the middle of nowhere with my soul mate with paws, but I did not exploit my canine's inexperience or small size in a dog-eat-dog world. We hiked onward in the dark to a truck stop.

A scruffy, gray-haired diesel truck driver wearing a cowboy hat asked me if we wanted anything in the café. I mumbled, "Iced tea with lemon—water for my pup." The man returned with a large tea and lemon slices in hand and gave my dog water. The driver was headed to

Miami and his invite to join him was accepted. It was the best lemon-sweetened tea in my life, and I felt at home.

THE HISTORY OF LEMONS

The lemon (*Citrus lemon*) is not a new superfood. The powerful oval-shaped canary-yellow superfruit can be traced back to the beginning of time. Lemons are believed to have first been used in India or China. Then, the citrus fruit entered Europe, near Italy during the time of ancient Rome, and we know that lemons were enjoyed in both the Arab world and the Mediterranean region between 1000 and 1150 A.D. There are also records of lemons being cultivated and grown in Genoa in the 1400s. Later, it is believed that the explorer Christopher Columbus brought lemon seeds on voyages and used lemons for medicinal purposes.

Also, it is a known fact that sailors on ships would use the versatile lemon for its vitamin C content, which helped stave off disease. In 1747, James Linds observed seamen suffering from scurvy (a disease linked to a lack of vitamin C that results in swollen, bleeding gums and open wounds that do not heal). He added lemon juice to their diets, and by the end of the eighteenth century scurvy was no longer the scourge of sailors.

SUPER NUTRIENTS

Lemons contain antioxidants, such as phytochemicals, polyphenols, tannins, and terpenes. The fruit, juice, rind, and zest all include nutritional value, too. As noted, lemons are a super source of the antioxidant vitamin C. Plus, this superfruit is low in calories, fat, and sodium, so this healthful and a diet-friendly superfruit can be used in appetizers, entrees, desserts, salads, smoothies, and beverages.

HEALTH BENEFITS OF LEMONS

Oranges, not lemons, are often the number-one superfruit in other superfoods books and articles. But the tart lemon, a cleansing fruit, is gaining attention, and there are many reasons why it's a superstar in

Superfoodsland. Lemon rind contains flavonoids, which help your arteries stay healthy and unclogged and keep heart attacks and strokes at bay. But the lemon is a cancer-fighting superfruit, too. Lemon peels contain two compounds—limonoids and limonene—both touted for their ability to help stave off different cancers. And another limonoid, called limonin, may help to lower levels of "bad" LDL cholesterol.[1]

Lemons do much more. New York–based Fred Pescatore, M.D., M.P.H., points out the healing powers of lemons: "They help alkalize your body, which lowers inflammation and disease." Medical research shows inflammation is often linked to a variety of chronic and acute ailments and even to cancer and heart disease.

The Legend of Limeys

Centuries ago, maritime seamen explored the Indian and Pacific Oceans. Crew members fought scurvy (a disease caused by a lack of vitamin C). The Portuguese explorer Vasco da Gama lost countless men to the disease while in route to India in the 1500s. Later on, Captain James Cook, from England, made his crew eat sauerkraut with lime juice. By 1800, lime juice was given to sailors in the Royal Navy—and from this antidote British seamen are called "limeys."[2]

MORE CITRUS SUPERFRUITS

I chose lemons as my favorite citrus fruit, but that doesn't mean other citrus fruits aren't nutritious or superfoods.

Grapefruit (*Citrus paradise*): Once called a "forbidden fruit," this citrus delight contains phytochemicals and lycopene and is a source of vitamin C, which are super nutrients to keep you heart-healthy and lower your risk of developing cancer.

Lime (*Rutaceae*): Like lemons and oranges, limes are liked for the tart flavor and used in infused water, cooking, and baking. This fruit contains plenty of vitamin C at 35 percent of your RDA, and its peel contains polyphenols and terpenes. It is helpful for preventing dermatitis as well as gum issues.

Orange (*Citrus sinensis*): This popular superfood often gets more attention than lemons and for good reason. It contains vitamin C, like its yellow cousin, fiber, and potassium. The orange is excellent for enhancing the immune system.

It doesn't matter which citrus fruit or rind you use in your diet—all of them contain superfood nutrients. Mixing citrus fruits, much like mixing gelato and yogurt, provides more flavor and variety, like in this sweet and tangy smoothie that takes me back to Florida, a place where I experienced orange groves and the Keys. (See more of lemon's benefits in Chapter 25, "Home Remedies from Your Kitchen," and Chapter 26, "Beautifying Superfoods.")

Super Immune-Boosting Citrus Smoothie

In the mornings, before a busy day, blending up a super smoothie, like this one, is as good as it gets when you're craving energy and a quick, nutritious drink. This healthful smoothie doesn't boast a lot of strange ingredients, but it does contain basic sweet and tart foods to energize. Fresh fruits, including banana and lemon and orange juices, provide vitamin C for a super immune-boosting beverage. This recipe is mine and is inspired by my love for its superfoods—superfruit, Greek yogurt, ice cream, and other foods I've yet to introduce to you.

1 banana, frozen, peeled, diced

⅓ cup Greek vanilla yogurt

½ cup premium vanilla ice cream

⅓ cup organic 2-percent milk

3 tablespoons fresh-squeezed orange juice

> 2 tablespoons fresh-squeezed lemon juice
>
> 5 ice cubes, crushed
>
> 2 tablespoons almonds, chopped fine
>
> 1 teaspoon raw honey or maple syrup
>
> 1 teaspoon pure vanilla extract
>
> ¼ teaspoon cinnamon
>
> Dash of nutmeg
>
> Fresh mint
>
> In a blender, mix all ingredients until creamy and thick. Add flavoring. Pour into a milkshake glass. Sprinkle with nutmeg. Garnish with mint. Use a straw or long spoon.
>
> Makes 2 servings.

So, it's time to put the lemons back in a dish on the kitchen counter and take out a surprising superfood from your kitchen cupboard. Hello, maple syrup. In the next chapter, I'll tout this health food—it's time. People in the northeastern United States and Canada know exactly why the maple leaf and syrup are sacred, but if you're skeptical, read on to get the latest scoop on nature's sweetener.

SUPER-IOR HEALING SUPERFOODS FOR THOUGHT

✓ Lemons (and other citrus fruits) may help lower the risk of developing cancers, reduce levels of bad cholesterol, boost immunity, and much more.

✓ Antioxidant-rich lemons and their powers are recognized around the world as healing medicines.

✓ Lemons, not unlike their counterparts grapefruits and oranges, heal in a variety of ways—thanks to their amazing properties.

✓ Lemons and their rind can help aid your body from head to toe.

Maple Syrup

Maple-trees are the cows of trees (spring-milked).
—HENRY WARD BEECHER

After experiencing the Deep South, with its southern hospitality, grits, and hominy, I trekked up north. One of my favorite superfoods, prevalent in the Northeast, is maple syrup. It was a reminder of my roots in California. Here's why. Coming back to the United States when crossing the Quebec-Vermont border was an unforgettable experience. When I had ended up in Montreal at dusk I had suffered a megabout of cultural shock. Like Dorothy in the land of Oz, neither I nor my little dog with a brave heart was prepared for the intensity of a foreign land.

In Vermont, the vibrant-colored maple trees of the fall welcomed us with their hues of reds, oranges, and yellows. Another truck driver we rode with spoke of harvesting fruits and vegetables, of farms and pumpkin patches. We stopped at a roadside café. He looked at me, the hippie girl from the West Coast, and he said, "You look like you could use a hot meal." I was treated to a plate of hotcakes with Vermont maple syrup. The taste of sweet syrup brought me back to the Sunday breakfasts my mother used to make, and I was grateful for being back home in the United States, one state over the line.

THE HISTORY OF MAPLE SYRUP

Maple syrup historians give credit for the development of maple syrup to the squirrel, a creature seen burrowing in the maple trees. It is also believed that American Indians of the Ottawa River valley noted maple sap as a source of super energy and nutrition. Others claim the local people of the northeastern region of North America have harvested sap for the production of maple syrup for centuries. When European settlers arrived in North America, they introduced the colonists to the maple syrup process, which entails tapping the trunks of maples to harvest the sap. Since then, many farmers in the northeastern region of the United States have made syrup for personal use and for sale.

By the 1900s, maple syrup was used throughout the United States, mostly as a topping for pancakes and waffles. These days, maple syrup is paired with other superfoods, such as granola, ice cream, oatmeal, smoothies, and sweet potatoes.

In the twenty-first century, the French-Canadian province of Quebec is the largest producer (70 percent of the world's supply of maple syrup), and Vermont is the biggest producer in the United States, according to food historians and maple syrup experts.

SUPER NUTRIENTS

While honey is touted as one of nature's top superfood sweeteners, premium antioxidant-rich maple syrup is getting more recognition for its nutritional benefits. It's finally getting noticed by some nutritionists, medical studies show the proof of its compounds, and maple syrup is even considered a "new" superfood—and for good reason, a lot of them, actually.

One-fourth cup of premium maple syrup contains fewer calories than high-fructose corn syrup, honey, or brown sugar. It boasts more calcium, manganese, magnesium, potassium, riboflavin, and zinc than most sweeteners. That means, overall, that maple syrup has more nutritional perks than other sweeteners. And there's more.

Maple syrup has more disease-fighting antioxidants than raw cabbage, tomatoes, and cantaloupe—also superfoods. So, it's no surprise maple syrup made its way on the top 20 superfoods list. Caveat: Classification of syrup matters (much like honey) and it's the Grade A type you want to be including in your diet.

Tapping into the Maple Trees

Maple syrup, according to the people who work for the Crown Maple syrup company, "it's not just for pancakes," and as a superfood fan and nature-loving tree lover, I agree. Take a journey with me into the winter wonderland of tapping time in the Hudson River valley, straight from the hardworking folks at Crown Maple.

"One of the exciting times of the year for us at Crown Maple is the tapping season. We typically start in January when winter has traditionally taken hold in our maple forest and put it into a deep, cold slumber. We rise ahead of the sun and gather our gear, and warm clothes, to hit the mountain as the sun begins to show its shining face.

"With more than 150,000 taps, we must properly plan our attack of the maple forest, proceeding section by section, branch line by branch line. Our network of tubing is all in place and each maple already has a dormant drop line waiting an opportunity to come to life. We approach the maple tube, give it a rub, and identify where previous holes are, as we make sure not to tap in the same areas. With our power drill, we put a 5/16-inch hole in the tree, we then hammer in the tap, and attach the tube that has been patiently waiting since the end of last season.

"If the day is warm, we will already be able to take a taste of the maple sap. It is clean, and cool, looks and tastes like water, hardly able to taste the two percent sugar. One tap done, 149,99 to go."

HEALTH BENEFITS OF MAPLE SYRUP

We know tapping maple trees is hard work, but the health virtues of maple syrup are worth it. Medical studies abound that show maple syrup, thanks to its multiple ingredients, may help lower your risk of heart disease and enhance your immune system, which means fewer colds and flu, and perhaps even lower odds of infection from bacteria. Here's proof.

Scientists discovered that polyphenol extract from the new superfood maple syrup may be just what you need to keep yourself from having to take a dose of prescription antibiotics. As revealed in the medical journal *Applied and Environmental Microbiology*, maple syrup works like an antibiotic and may prevent bacteria from affecting your immune system and causing an infection.[1]

Also, scientists at Quebec's Université Laval discovered an anti-inflammation molecule and published their findings in *Bioorganic & Medicinal Chemistry Letters*. Credit is given to quebecol, which is formed during the process of making maple syrup, and it may even aid in staving off the inflammation process in diseases like rheumatoid arthritis.[2]

Maple Syrup on the Brain

In the summer of 2017, I traveled to Victoria, British Columbia (a place, like Quebec City, I always wanted to experience but hesitated because it was outside my comfort zone). I appreciated a variety of superfoods there, from cheese plates to heirloom tomatoes. It was a special superfood, of sorts, that had me at the words "made with real maple syrup." At Victoria International Airport, in a gift shop, I was drawn to the food items aisle. A box of Canadian-produced maple leaf cookies caught my eye.

Once back home, when I settled in, it was time. As I printed out my photos, from the tearoom at the Fairmont Hotel to Fisherman's Wharf and the seal that greeted me to the boat ride on the Gorge, I treated myself to a pot of brewed tea paired with the Canadian maple leaf cookies infused with maple syrup. This teatime took me back to Victoria. You can order imported Canadian maple leaf cookies online, or order maple leaf cookie cutters and create cookies using superfoods like whole-grain flour, eggs, maple syrup, and maple sugar. Also, using maple syrup in different ways, like a maple syrup–infused salad dressing, may give you that northern connection.

Also, chocolate can be infused with real maple syrup from Vermont. Pairing the two superfoods is a sweet experience. But syrup can also be enjoyed in wholesome dishes like a spinach salad.

Super Cleansing Strawberry and Spinach Salad with Miso-Maple Dressing

What exactly is the flavor of miso? Enjoyed by itself, the first reaction you might have is pure umami, but when blended with maple syrup and a light vinegar, miso binds with them into a dressing that delivers a gentle, creamy sweetness without overwhelming the other ingredients. Add a handful of spinach, some sliced strawberries, and some candied nuts, and you've got a great, colorful salad for lunch or dinner.

For the dressing

¼ cup olive oil
1 tablespoon white miso
1 tablespoon maple syrup
   (Crown Maple, amber
   color, rich taste)

1 tablespoon white wine
   vinegar or rice wine
   vinegar
Kosher salt and freshly
   ground black pepper,
   to taste

For the salad

1 cup sliced almonds
1 tablespoon maple sugar
   (Crown Maple)
6 cups baby spinach

1 cup sliced strawberries
6–12 long strips shaved
   Parmesan

Combine all the dressing ingredients (except salt and pepper) in a clean jar with a lid. Seal the jar and shake the dressing until it is fully emulsified and creamy. Taste the dressing and season with salt and pepper to your liking, then set aside.

Toast the almonds in a hot dry pan over medium heat until just fragrant, about 5 minutes. Sprinkle the maple sugar over the nuts. Remove the pan from the heat and stir to coat with the maple sugar while the nuts are still warm.

Put the spinach in a large bowl, gently add the strawberries on top. Add the almonds, drizzle half of the dressing over the top, and toss to lightly coat. Add the remainder of the dressing just before serving, and garnish with the strips of Parmesan. (Any leftover dressing can be kept in the sealed container in the refrigerator for up to 1 week.)

(Courtesy: Crown Maple and *The Crown Maple Guide to Maple Syrup*)

Now that you are looking at your maple syrup with approval, come with me to the next superfoods. Much like maple syrup, the next ones are not to be overlooked, either. Living in the Golden State—a hub for nuts—there's a lot to share and to explain about what makes nuts versatile superfoods.

SUPER-IOR HEALING SUPERFOODS FOR THOUGHT

✓ Maple syrup may help lower the risk of developing cancers, reduce levels of bad cholesterol, boost immunity, and much more.

✓ Maple syrup and its healing powers are approved by researchers, especially in Canada and the northeastern United States, where the superfood is prevalent.

✓ Maple syrup heals in a variety of ways—thanks to its antioxidants and other amazing properties.

✓ As one of nature's finest sweeteners, like honey, maple syrup deserves to be noticed in the land of superfoods.

✓ Using maple syrup with other superfoods, including superfruits and supergrains, provides a lot of healing powers.

11

Nuts and Nutty Butters

Mellow nuts have the hardest rind.
—SIR WALTER SCOTT

Wandering across America came with a mixed bag of superfoods, hot and cold; it was either feast or famine. I found myself in a small mom-and-pop store somewhere in the Midwest. Again, I was penniless but with a new knapsack and sleeping bag. As luck would have it, at dusk, the son was tending the store. He was fascinated with my nomadic lifestyle with a dog. As I answered his questions about life on the road, he said I could choose any foods I wanted to fill my knapsack. I felt like I won a lottery, and I scurried around the aisles to find superfoods: Nuts (peanuts to cashews) were on my list, and a large jar of nutty peanut butter was definitely put on the countertop, making me feel like I was back home with familiar foods.

As a kid, I remember that on the dining room table (especially during autumn and the holiday season) there was often a wooden bowl full of mixed nuts, including almonds and walnuts—my two favorite nuts. It took longer to crack, shell, and eat these crunchy nuggets, but it was fun. And these days, while my nut repertoire has expanded, I still favor almonds and walnuts. These versatile wonders were familiar to me a few years ago when I purchased the dark chocolate–covered almonds found in bins at grocery stores.

The roots of California almonds, however, go way back before my time. The facts are fascinating, and I want to expound on the almond since I'm from the West Coast state touted for its almonds—more than 75 percent of the world's supply comes from Central California. I'm dedicating the nuts chapter to the almond, but I'll certainly dish out information on other nuts that may be your favorites.

THE HISTORY OF ALMONDS

The beginning of the almond tree seems to have different stories, but it may be that it first grew in Asia. It is believed that almonds were a survival food for explorers while traveling the Silk Road going from Asia to the Mediterranean. Some food historians believe that almond trees were first planted in California in the mid-1700s, giving credit to Spanish Franciscan padres. While the almond tree didn't grow well in the coastal regions, it did blossom in the Central Valley due to its fertile ground.[1]

SUPER NUTRIENTS

The almond isn't really a nut (although we call it that); it's a fruit called a drupe, as are cherries, plums, and olives. It's an ancestor of stone fruits, and it's nutritious. Almonds are low in saturated fat, contain no cholesterol, and boast plenty of dietary fiber. Also, don't forget this nut also contains calcium, potassium, and protein.

Almonds also supply energy and are low in saturated fat. They are an excellent source of the antioxidant vitamin E and magnesium. With a super nutritional lineup like this, it's no super surprise that nuts are considered a superfood.[2]

In a large study, more than seventeen thousand children and adults changed their snack habits by incorporating nuts such as almonds. The findings were that their diet changed into a more healthful one thanks to substituting almonds; it led to a more nutrient-dense diet with fewer empty calories and less sodium and more good fat.[3]

HEALTH BENEFITS OF ALMONDS

Almonds are an excellent source of monounsaturated fat, which gives them the label of being heart-healthy. While they do have other nutrients, the good fat content makes these nuts stand out. Since nuts are rich in disease-fighting antioxidants and a plethora of nutrients, it's no surprise they can lower your risk for heart disease and may help stave off Alzheimer's disease, type 2 diabetes, and cancer. There's also research that nuts may help reduce inflammatory diseases such as asthma and rheumatoid arthritis.[4]

SUPER HEALING POWERS OF OTHER NUTS

Medical doctors and researchers have discovered a handful of nuts can lower your risk of developing heart disease, cancer, and even type 2 diabetes, thanks to those "good" monounsaturated fats (like what's found in olive oil). Read on to see all of what nuts may do for you.

SUPER NUTTY BUTTERS

You may favor peanut butter, a popular nutty delight, but there are other types of nutty butters just like there are other kinds of nuts. Nut butters, including almond, cashew, and hazelnut (creamy, nutty, and even infused with honey) can help make smoothies creamier, cookies tastier, sandwiches more delicious, and they can do much more, too. Not only do nut butters taste super, they also are nutritious and can be used in granolas, cookies, and sandwiches—and eaten by the spoonful.

Back in my early twenties, when I hitchhiked with Tiger, my first road canine companion, a Lhasa Apso/Maltese mix dog (who broke my heart when he was stolen later in Las Vegas, Nevada, ironically outside of Lady Luck Casino), across America and up in to Canada, we were stranded at night on a busy road. Nobody could see us to snag a ride, so I made the decision to sleep in the forest. After settling in our sleeping bag, I took out a jar of peanut butter and a plastic spoon. It was our nighttime snack. I felt lonely but content: I was filled up with the creamy nut butter, cuddled up with my best friend, and surrounded by trees with my dream of making it over the border the next day.

TOP 10 SUPER NUTS

Type	Superfood Nutrients	May Help Lower Risk
Almonds	High in flavonoids and vitamin E, fiber, monounsaturated fat, zinc	Alzheimer's disease, heart disease, diabetes
Brazil Nuts	Rich in selenium, a mineral that, like vitamin E, is a disease-fighting antioxidant	Cancer
Cashews	High in monounsaturated fat, copper, magnesium, and protein; no cholesterol	Heart disease
Hazelnuts	Vitamin E, oleic acid, phenols	Heart disease
Macadamia Nuts	Rich in monounsaturated fat	Heart disease, obesity
Peanuts	Boast niacin and folate—two B vitamins	Cancer, mental disorders
Pecans	Antioxidants, monounsaturated fat	Cancer, heart disease
Pine Nuts	Rich in monounsaturated fat	Heart disease
Pistachios	Phytosterols	Cancer, heart disease, high levels of HDL ("bad") cholesterol
Walnuts	Rich in omega-3 fatty acids	Heart disease

(Source: *The Healing Powers of Chocolate* by Cal Orey)

When you have creature comforts (including a kitchen with cooking aids), making your own nut butter is easy. Years later in my mountain cabin (dog and trees included), I did just that. After purchasing a jar of a nondescript brand of almond butter, I decided I could make a better nut butter myself. All you do is put shelled nuts in a blender or food processor, add honey if you'd like, a bit of olive or canola oil, sea salt (optional), and blend until creamy. Yes, it works! Then, store the butter into an airtight plastic container and put it into the refrigerator. However, premade nut butters are available in supermarkets and health food stores, and you can purchase different kinds online.

So, we've got almonds, the nut I chose as number one, other nuts, and the world of super nutty butters. People tell me the almond is not their favorite nut because it's too hard to eat. The thing is, I do agree (but I still munch on dark-chocolate-covered almonds). Still, almonds come in countless forms. Almonds can be found in the shell (to be cracked like I did when I was a kid raiding the wooden bowl full of nuts), blanched, and sliced (found in the baking aisle at a supermarket), and as almond confections, yogurt-coated almonds (I used to find these at grocery store bins), almond paste, almond milk, and almond oil.

And you can use the variety of forms listed above in countless dishes, including dips, snack mixes, salads, stir-fry dishes, pasta plates, poultry and fish entrees, and no-cook desserts such as energy bars and balls. The almond is truly a versatile superfood.

Super Invigorating Almond Butter Energy Truffles

❖ ❖ ❖

When did this popular, candy-rich, no-bake bite appear? It may have started during the health-oriented tofu-and-granola craze in the seventies. But it also is a spin-off of no-bake cookies infused with alcohol that go back to the mid-twentieth century. So, here is a version of my get-up-and-go energy balls. What's better than bite-sized balls with wholesome goodness that are easy to make from nature's finest superfoods. And they contain healthful protein from the nuts and nut butter, energizing carbs, fiber, and iron.

1 cup creamy almond butter (or peanut butter)
⅓ cup honey
⅓ cup premium unsweetened cocoa powder
½ cup walnuts, chopped
¼ cup golden raisins

1 cup premium sweetened coconut flakes
2 teaspoons sea salt
Cinnamon and ginger, to taste

In a large bowl, combine nut butter, honey, and cocoa powder. Stir well. Fold in walnuts and raisins. Put into refrigerator for about 30 minutes. (This makes it easier to make the balls.) Shape into 2-inch balls, roll in coconut. Sprinkle with salt and spices. Store balls in airtight container. You can also switch it up and use different dried fruit, like the superfruits blueberries and cranberries.

The different colors and textures of these energy bites are pleasing to the eye and palate. They are gooey, chewy, and crunchy. Plus, the mix of nuts and honey with a bit of sea salt gives you both a sweet and savory super treat. And the spices give these bites a brilliant note.

Makes about 1 dozen truffles.

Take a break with an energy ball or two and continue on the journey in Superfoodsland. Give the next superfood pick a warm welcome. I'll show you how pasta—a dieters' forbidden food—is one more "new" (and versatile) superfood on my favorites list, if you choose the right kind.

SUPER-IOR HEALING SUPERFOODS FOR THOUGHT

✓ Nuts contain good-for-you monounsaturated fat, which can be heart-healthy if eaten in moderation.

✓ Almonds, like a variety of other antioxidant-rich nuts, can help lower your risk of developing heart disease and cancer.

✓ Pairing nuts with other superfoods, including apples, berries, leafy greens, and Greek yogurt, gives you crunchy texture, flavor, and more antioxidants, minerals, and vitamins.

✓ Salted nuts can be a trigger food, like potato chips, so to keep it healthy, eat only a handful of nuts each day, and the lightly salted or no-salt varieties are your best bet.

Pasta (Whole Grain)

*No man is lonely while eating spaghetti: it requires
so much attention.*
—CHRISTOPHER MORLEY

In the late seventies, an era of trail-mix devotees, pasta wasn't ignored
on the list of fitness foods. As hippie girls, like me, went back to
school, to make our lives easier, the Crock-Pot came to the rescue.
One afternoon my mate put together a homemade red sauce for
spaghetti. (My job was to bring the pasta home.) I arrived late with
whole-grain noodles and vegetables for a French-style pasta prima-
vera—not the traditional white spaghetti and meatballs we used to
love. I boiled the pasta and added the vegetables, looking in horror at
the hamburger in the pot. (Think pet rabbit boiling in *Fatal Attraction.*) As a *Kramer vs. Kramer*–like scene of a man and woman not seeing eye-to-eye chill filled the room, it was the beginning of a parting of
the ways.

As a grad student, I embraced whole-grain bagels and granola at the
student union, while my mate's idea of lunchtime pasta favorites was
canned SpaghettiOs, an American round-shaped pasta in a cheese-
and-tomato soup. It was a *Days of Wine and Roses* food-style breakup,
and I moved on to explore Superfoodsland. On the upside, pasta (lin-

guini, fettuccine, shell, and bow-tie—all whole grain) became a frequent superfood in my life of singledom (with a dog in tow). And years later, I welcomed a variety of pasta plates, from linguini with clam sauce to vegetarian lasagna.

THE HISTORY OF PASTA

It's no wonder that the roots of pasta come from Italy, a country touted for its sinful spaghetti to live for. Some European food historians (not just one) will share with you (most likely over a plate of pasta) that by the eighteenth century, Italians had discovered the ways of mass production, so there was no need to make fresh pasta in the kitchen—the way some chefs do to get super praise on a Food Network TV show during the food challenge segments.

SUPER NUTRIENTS

A 2-ounce serving (about 1 cup cooked pasta) has almost no fat, 200 calories, some protein, and enough potassium, calcium, iron, and niacin to make it a supergrain, especially if it's whole grain.

What's more, this type of pasta is higher in fiber than the white, so it's more filling. That means you will eat less but feel more satisfied eating the super stuff, such as flat strands of fettuccine, spiral-shaped rotini, and long linguini, plus dozens of other varieties of shapes and sizes of the nutritious superfood.

Not only is pasta (eaten in moderation) a heart-healthy, nutritious food when paired with other nutrient-dense superfoods, including cheese, cruciferous vegetables, leafy greens, poultry, shellfish, and tomato sauce, but you also get a super heart-healthy dish.

HEALTH BENEFITS OF PASTA

Surprise! You *can* enjoy the high complex-carbohydrate content of whole-grain pasta, which may be partially responsible for its ability to help keep blood sugar levels on an even keel, stave off type 2 diabetes, and much more.

Past research shows that in Mediterranean countries, such as Italy and France, where indulging in pasta is not shunned, the risk of developing heart disease is lower than in other countries. One reason may be that a high-carb diet, versus one high in fat, lowers the risk of heart disease, including clogged arteries.

Not only is pasta heart-healthy, it's also energizing, not fattening. For years, while I have been making, ordering, and eating pasta—all shapes and sizes, paired with plant-based foods—friends and family say, "No thanks, pasta can pack on the pounds." This is not true, and now there's proof!

A study of more than twenty-three thousand Italian people (not lab rats) was part of the revelation that pasta is a good-for-you, slimming superfood. The people were given a questionnaire regarding what and how much each person had eaten the previous day. The results: The volunteers who had eaten pasta were found to be lean, not overweight. The findings, published in the journal *Nutrition and Diabetes*, reveal intriguing facts. Eating pasta was found to link to better weight management when it is part of the Mediterranean diet. What's more, pasta contributes to a healthy body-mass index (lower waist circumference and ideal waist-hip ratio). So, the authors of the breakthrough research project gave a thumbs-up to pasta.[1]

If you enjoy creamy cheese sauces with pasta, remember less is more, and in moderation you can enjoy them. But using tomato-rich sauces, homemade, can make your pasta eating even more superfood rich, especially paired with cheese and/or vegetables.

Cannelloni

I love cooking pasta (it's easy to do, plop it in a pan and boil) and pairing it with superfoods. These days, we don't overcook and simmer for hours and hours. Al dente pasta and a variety of crisp vegetables provide superfood perks. So, here are two easy, down-to-earth recipes inspired by the former San Carlos, California's Salvatore's Italian restaurant owner-chef—two favorites of mine.

For the homemade sauce

1 tablespoon olive oil
1 tablespoon garlic, minced
6 tablespoons organic tomato paste

1 cup water
2 tablespoons herbs, fresh or dried, including basil, thyme
Black pepper, to taste

For the cannelloni

½ box cannelloni, whole grain
1 tablespoon olive oil
1 clove garlic, minced
2 tablespoons herbs, fresh or dried
1 cup fresh spinach, chopped

2-3 Roma tomatoes, chopped
1 cup ricotta cheese mixed with homemade sauce
4–5 slices mozzarella
Fresh Parmesan, grated

In a skillet, heat oil over medium heat. Add garlic. Add tomatoes, paste, and water. Stir. Heat to a boil. Add herbs and pepper. Simmer for a few minutes. Set aside. In a saucepan, cook pasta. In a skillet, heat olive oil with garlic. Add herbs. Mix spinach and tomatoes with the ricotta mixture and add oil and garlic. Fill the pasta. Place in a baking dish with half of the sauce on the bottom. Drizzle homemade sauce on top of the pasta. Top with mozzarella. Bake at 350 degrees F, about 30 minutes. Top with grated Parmesan.

This dish is as good as it gets. The different cheeses and chunks of vegetables will remind you that you're eating fresh superfoods.

Super Energizing One-Power Bowl Pasta with Vegetables

❖ ❖ ❖

As a kid, on weekdays, I didn't mind eating Kraft Mac & Cheese from a box. But on Sunday, it was a day to celebrate. Homemade sauce topped on linguini and paired with fresh vegetables got rave reviews from my family and me. Nowadays, we can have our pasta and eat it too (any day of the week). And time isn't a factor.

2 cups whole-grain rotini (Eden Spinach Spirals)

2 cups fresh vegetable mix (broccoli, cauliflower, tomatoes, wild mushrooms), washed, chopped

2 teaspoons fresh garlic, minced

2 teaspoons onion, chopped

2 tablespoons extra-virgin olive oil

1 teaspoon European-style butter

Ground pepper and sea salt, to taste

Parmesan, shavings

Pine nuts, to taste

¼ cup fresh basil, chopped

Follow cooking pasta instructions (7–8 minutes, al dente) on the package, using water. While pasta cooks, stir-fry vegetable mix, garlic, and onion in oil and butter. Add pepper and salt. Top cooked pasta with vegetables. Lightly toss. Combine pasta and vegetables equally in individual serving bowls. Top each with cheese, nuts, and basil. Pair with slices of artisanal whole-grain French bread or a baguette dipped in olive oil or spread with a bit of butter.

Makes 3–4 servings.

We agree super pasta is a superfood, right? So, now you'll be more apt to embrace the next superfood! I'll show you how pizza (a fatty food that can be good for you!), much like pasta (without thick, creamy sauces and meat), is a "new" superfood that doesn't get the credit it deserves. It's known that pizza is a favorite food, but it's the ingredients used that can convert it to a superfood.

SUPER-IOR HEALING SUPERFOODS FOR THOUGHT

✓ Pasta may help lower the risk of developing cancers, reduce levels of bad cholesterol, boost immunity, and much more.

✓ Pasta and its healing powers are recognized around the world as healing medicines.

✓ Whole-grain pasta, not unlike other good carbs, heals in a variety of ways—thanks to its antioxidants and other amazing properties.

✓ When paired with other superfoods, including cheese, crucifers, and tomatoes, whole-grain pasta is a superfood that is popular in countless countries and the United States, too.

Pizza (with Toppings)

*You better cut the pizza in four pieces because I'm
not hungry enough to eat six.*
—YOGI BERRA

If you've mastered the art of eating wholesome pasta (with or without
a mate), pizza will be a piece of cake, if you listen up. In my thirties, I
graduated college and entered the world of freelancing as a magazine
journalist. One weekend, I was on assignment to interview homeless
people and their dogs. I traveled to Berkeley, a place of serious, health-
conscious foodies.

After interviews with down-and-out people, young and old, I
stopped at my pet pizza spot. The Italian café, always busy, made the
best whole-wheat crust vegetarian pizza. Once served, I ate a few
pieces and was in superfood heaven. When I left the diner, a middle-
aged man and his German shepherd were panhandling for spare
change. I offered my doggie box of pizza, but the man wanted money.
I gave both in exchange for an interview. In hindsight, I'm reminded
of Will Smith in *I Am Legend*, when he told his German shepherd,
Sam, to eat her vegetables. And I wanted to pay it forward like the person in Vermont did for me with hotcakes and maple syrup.

THE HISTORY OF PIZZA

Welcome to pizza, a timeless favorite, and in my world it's a superfood. Pizza is believed to have been introduced and enjoyed as far back as 6000 B.C. The Italian food was allegedly consumed by Egyptians, Greeks, and Romans.

Food historians will share with you that in Naples during the 1700s and 1800s, pizza was a food popular with money-challenged folks. The food was called "flat breads," and it had a lot of different toppings. Some of these flat breads eaten by the poor in Naples were topped with cheese and tomatoes—two superfoods on the top 20 list in this book.

The first pizza place to make its name in America was Lombardi's in New York City, which opened in 1905. And then pizza lovers helped pave the way to the pizza craze of the twentieth century, which is still going strong in the twenty-first century. But it is whole-grain crust and superfood toppings that make it a healthful food.

Super Pizza Pie for Royalty

Yes, pizza does have roots. It isn't just a fast food to pick up at a pizza parlor or the frozen food aisle at your supermarket. It used to be a royal treat. Food historians share the tale of King Umberto and Queen Margherita of Italy, who visited Naples in the late 1800s. As the legend goes, the royal couple were bored with French cuisine and requested pizza from the city's popular pizza hub. It is said the queen favored white cheese, tomatoes, and basil. As time passed, this cheese pizza was named Pizza Margherita.

SUPER NUTRIENTS

Yes, a slice of pizza can be super nutritious—as long as you order vegetable and cheese toppings. The crust—if whole wheat—gives you lots of energy and a dose of more good-for-you nutrients. Choose superfood cheeses, such as goat cheese, feta, Parmesan, or aged cheddar, to provide you with extra calcium and protein perks. Not to forget a tomato-based (or basil-rich pesto) sauce. Fat count: 6 to 12 grams per slice.

HEALTH BENEFITS OF PIZZA

What is delicious, cheesy with toppings, and may help lower your risk of developing cancer and heart disease? Pizza! I'm not dishing up a deep dish, super cheesy, pepperoni-laden pie, mind you; I'm talking about a healthful pie. Years ago, when I was a health magazine journalist, an assignment on healing foods was given to me. It was my job to think outside of the box, and I added pizza because of its cancer-fighting lycopene-rich tomato sauce. And medical research backed up this delicious superfood that I added on to my article. Here's proof.

According to a study reported by the *International Journal of Cancer*, Italian researchers found that regular eating of pizza could help lower the risk of developing different cancers. It seems that following a traditional Mediterranean diet could be a factor, too, and that includes adding olive oil and tomatoes—two ingredients often included in a healthful pizza.[1]

But how can superfood tomatoes on pizza and in pizza sauce be cancer fighting? In a pizza pie, it's like this: Rich in the antioxidant lycopene, tomatoes may lower the risk of prostate and colon cancers by preventing damage caused by harmful molecules called free radicals, which contribute to cancer.

Eating pizza slices every day is not advised, nor is daily drinking of green smoothies, as the characters do in the Hallmark Channel film *Like Cats and Dogs*. In that movie, the uptight cat-lover Spencer is following a strict raw-food diet, including dark beet juice, whereas Lara, a fun and spontaneous dog lover, favors pizza for breakfast (and s'mores for a snack). The polar opposites end up incorporating both superfoods—and each other—into their lives. The motto: Adding a balance of favorite superfoods into your life can be a good thing.

Super Satisfying Pacific Northwest Veggie Pesto Pizza

❖ ❖ ❖

After one Bellevue, Washington, book signing at a Barnes and Noble bookstore, I was hungry and didn't want to be in a busy restaurant. Back in my hotel room, with a balcony view to cherish, I scanned the pricey room service menu. I ordered a take-out pizza. The ten-inch whole-wheat crusted pick included mozzarella cheese, artichokes, roasted red pepper, portobello mushrooms, spinach, sun-dried tomatoes, caramelized onions, and feta cheese. It was delivered from pizza heaven and made my stay feel like home away from home.

1 store-bought, premade, premium, whole-wheat pizza crust

½ cup store-bought all-natural pesto sauce

½ cup cheese (feta or mozzarella)

½ cup each fresh spinach and kale, chopped

¼ cup heirloom, Roma, or sun-dried tomatoes, chopped

¼ cup fresh mango or pineapple, chopped in cubes

1 teaspoon fresh Italian seasoning

Olive oil (drizzle to taste)

¼ cup pine nuts

2 tablespoons fresh Parmesan, grated

On a baking sheet, place pizza crust with sauce, feta cheese, vegetables, and fruit. Add seasoning and oil. Bake at 400 degrees F until cheese melts and crust is toasted. You can place raw spinach and tomatoes on top like a fresh salad if preferred. Drizzle with oil, add nuts and Parmesan. Cut in slices.

Makes 4 servings.

If you're sold on the healing powers of pizza, poultry as a superfood should be an easy sell. Read on—discover why those chicken chunks in your soup or turkey slices on a whole-grain roll may be super good for you and good enough to say no to red meat.

SUPER-IOR HEALING SUPERFOODS FOR THOUGHT

✓ Whole-grain vegetarian pizza, not unlike other superfoods, heals in a variety of ways, thanks to its disease-fighting antioxidants, and paired with other amazing superfoods, it's a super superfood.

✓ Tomatoes and tomato sauce, usually found in pizza ingredients, are lycopene-rich, which means they can help lower the risk of developing different types of cancers.

✓ Indulging in a thin, whole-wheat crust, cutting the cheese content in half, and piling on an assortment of vegetables makes pizza a complete superfood meal.

✓ Trying different types of pizza with different types of cheese and tomatoes is not only an adventure for your palate but also provides a variety of healthful vitamins and minerals.

Poultry (Chicken/Turkey)

He was a blessing to all the juvenile part of the neighborhood, for in summer he was for ever forming parties to eat cold ham and chicken out of doors.
—JANE AUSTEN, *Sense and Sensibility*

After a decade of being a magazine journalist in the city, the mountain life greeted me, and I was now a health-and-nutrition book author. One winter afternoon, the deck was covered with heavy, wet snow. No birds—alive or cooked—were in sight. The pine trees and wires looked spooky shrouded with white powder. Not a stranger to power outages in the Sierra Nevada, I went into survival mode. I was clad in a hooded sweatshirt and jeans and felt like a character in a doomsday film as I took inventory of food. During the superstorm, since the gas had stayed on, I heated up my own soup that I had stashed for a rainy day in the freezer. The hearty soup for the soul was prepared with super-foods—chunks of white chicken breast, which can help make the challenge of a storm more bearable with its comforting taste. I can personally attest that the fragrance of herbs and garlic in the kitchen were amazing. While ready-made soups are quick and a godsend during power outages, having broth I made myself with TLC and added fresh superfood vegetables, including tomatoes, made a difference without the added sodium, and it just tastes, well, homemade.

Savoring the soup by a crackling fire (and praying that the lights don't go out) was worth writing home about. Nourishing the body, mind, and spirit with nature's finest ingredients during a storm, like that one, was not only comforting, it also ended up being a good omen. The lights stayed on, and I didn't catch the flu or the cold that was making its rounds.

THE HISTORY OF POULTRY

Food historians trace the eating of turkey and chicken back to the Stone Age era because they were wild game (all types of fowl) cavemen would hunt for food and survival. Throughout the centuries, both turkeys and chickens were hunted and eaten by cultures around the globe.

In the eighteenth century, farmers in the United States tended to chickens and made use of the birds and their edible eggs. By mid-nineteenth century, purchasing chicken and turkey at the supermarket and from the butcher was commonplace. Poultry was provided in a variety of ways, including in canned soups and frozen TV dinners, and in restaurants and cafes.

In the twenty-first century, the demand for cage-free, organic turkeys and chickens is growing because more consumers want to know the source of the bird and if it is free of hormones and antibiotics.

The Scoop on the First Turkey Feast

There are tales of pilgrims and turkey from the first Thanksgiving in 1621. As the story goes, the first colonists and Native Americans gathered at Plymouth Plantation in Massachusetts to celebrate a super feast after a good harvest season. This much is true, complete with an abundance of food. The catch is, some food historians insist turkey was not served until a few centuries later, but wild fowl like duck, goose, and stuffed birds were dished up. Wild turkeys were existent, but they weren't the centerpiece on the table to gobble up. Later, as history tells it, in a magazine called *Godey's Lady's Book*, a roast turkey recipe was shared. And in 1863, President Abraham Lincoln declared Thanksgiving, a.k.a, Turkey Day, a national holiday, complete with a turkey, which today is a touted superfood.

SUPER NUTRIENTS

Roasted turkey or chicken breast (without skin) is lower in fat than other commercial meats. That makes poultry like these two popular types an ideal superfood. Both birds contain plenty of minerals and B vitamins, aren't high in calories (especially the white meat), and are a good choice if you're watching your calories, cholesterol levels, and sodium numbers.

Superfood turkey also is rich in tryptophan. This compound helps your body make mood-boosting serotonin. Turkey is better than popping a happy pill and can not only calm your nerves with its vitamin B, but it's also a happy food.

Eating poultry is certainly part of the Mediterranean diet. The best chickens and turkeys come from a farm that allows free-range birds, raised on 100-percent vegetarian feed, with no antibiotics or preservatives. You can find this type of poultry at stores like Trader Joe's, your butcher, or on local farms.

Bone Broth—Warm Up to the Ancient Superfood

One day when I was at the hair salon, I overheard the stylists chatting about the newest diet rave—bone broth. As the *Healing Powers* series author, I was surprised by the broth since I hadn't heard about it. I did my homework and discovered bone broth is an ancient remedy that goes back to caveman era.

So, is chicken or turkey bone broth the new age soup for the soul and body? Perhaps, according to nutritionists like Robin Foroutan, R.D., who are hip to this broth—a superfood. Here's why. It's the collagen, says Foroutan. "It's an anti-aging superfood because it gives your body the building blocks it needs for skin, nail, hair, and joints," she points out. The nutritionist adds that collagen is a "super-glue" for your body from head to toe.

"The smell of homemade bone broth reminds me of my grandmother's house," she reminisces, adding that she cheats and buys the premade organic bone broth. "It's just as delicious and it's much faster." She adds spices such as turmeric, legumes such as white beans or lentils, and other vegetables. The reward: Foroutan sips super bone broth out of a mug to warm up and stay healthy on cold, winter days.

Homestyle-Bone Broth

Ann Louise Gittleman, Ph.D., C.N.S., also believes in the superpowers of bone broth. If you don't have the time to cook up a homemade batch, she recommends buying 100 percent organic bone broth. Here, is Gittleman's bone broth recipe; per my request, poultry is the protein source, rather than beef.

3 to 4 pounds of chicken or turkey bones	*3 celery sticks*
	2 medium yellow onions
1 tablespoon olive oil, avocado oil, or macadamia oil	*2 tablespoons cider vinegar*
	Water
2 medium carrots	*1 bay leaf*

Heat the oven to 400 degrees F. Place the bones on a baking tray and drizzle with olive oil. Place the tray in the oven, roasting the bones for 30 minutes. Turn the bones, then roast for another 30 minutes. Chop the carrots, celery, and onions roughly. You'll discard these after, so you don't need to be precise.

Place the roasted bones, chopped vegetables, bay leaf, and cider vinegar in a large stockpot. Cover with water so that the ingredients are under at least 2 inches of liquid. At this point, you can also add in other flavoring ingredients that you want into broth. Heat the broth over high heat until it comes to a rapid simmer, then reduce heat to low. Cover the broth and let it simmer on low for 12–24 hours. Skim off the foam from the top periodically. You may have to add water occasionally to make sure the ingredients stay covered. Strain and cool broth. After the broth has darkened to a rich brown color, remove it from the heat and strain through a fine-mesh sleeve.

Place the broth in a large container and let cool to room temperature. Once it's at room temperature, place it in the fridge to cool more and to store it. Scrape off any solidified fat that rises to the top before eating the broth. Reheat your bone broth for a steaming cup that you can sip on its own or use it as a powerful ingredient in your favorite recipes.

Enjoy several 8-ounce servings. (Soup quantity can vary, depending on the size of your ingredients.)

HEALTH BENEFITS OF POULTRY

White meat is lower in fat and calories, so it's a healthier choice than dark meat, whether you're consuming chicken or turkey. It's also good to know that medical researchers have found that it's free-range chickens (not grain-fed birds) that provide more omega-3 fatty acids (the good stuff that can maintain good heart health and keep your weight in check) and contain less harmful dietary fat.

Past medical research has also shown that chicken may lower your levels of "bad" cholesterol as well as help lower blood pressure. One serving of chicken contains less than 100 milligrams of cholesterol (our daily amount should be below 300 milligrams), so it can be a healthier choice of lean protein versus other meats. Choosing the healthiest poultry is important, too. In the twenty-first century, poultry-related words like *grass-fed, all natural, organic, no anti-*

biotics, *no preservatives*, and *oven-roasted* are things you want to hear from the butcher at the supermarket or another source of chicken and turkey.

Also, cooking poultry properly (not eating it undercooked) is the key to good health and to prevent gastrointestinal issues linked to E. coli or other bacterial woes. Pay attention to expiration dates and proper storage in the refrigerator at the right temperature. But overall, turkey is a superfood that is versatile, whether you make it the star on a holiday or enjoy it in a fresh salad.

Super Vitalizing Turkey Salad

❖ ❖ ❖

Turkey used in a salad should be an easy dish to put together. However, this recipe is chock-full of superfoods, from the ingredients in the salad to the dressing. The turkey bites are a celebration of cruciferous vegetables, tomatoes, superfruit, nuts, and lemon. It doesn't get better than this, so I chose to share this recipe with you.

For the salad

3 cups skinless, boneless, cooked turkey breasts, cut into bite-size pieces

1 pound cabbage, green or red, shredded

6 plum tomatoes, sliced across

4 green onions, thinly sliced

1½ cups fresh pineapple tidbits

2 beets, cooked, diced

¼ cup sesame, caraway, or poppy seeds

Sea salt and pepper, to taste

½ cup cashews, chopped

For the dressing

⅓ cup extra-virgin olive oil (Sciabica's or Marsala)

¼ cup lemon or lime juice

½ teaspoon oregano

2 tablespoons Dijon mustard

2 garlic cloves, minced

¼ cup parsley and/or basil, chopped

1 teaspoon curry powder

In large shallow serving bowl, combine turkey, cabbage, tomatoes, onions, pineapple, beets, seeds, salt, pepper, and cashews. Set aside. In a small bowl, whisk together oil, juice, oregano, mustard, garlic, parsley, and curry powder. Toss turkey mixture gently with dressing just before serving.

Makes 6 servings.

(Courtesy: Gemma Sanita Sciabica, from *Cooking with California Olive Oil: Recipes from the Heart for the Heart*)

Now that the superfoods chicken and turkey have made it to your must-have lean-protein list, it's back to a super vegetable. Next, I salute the potato. (In college, the potato bar with toppings was my favorite eating spot.) Take a look at why the super potato is another food that is, well, super.

SUPER-IOR HEALING SUPERFOODS FOR THOUGHT

✓ Eating chicken and turkey instead of red meat may help lower the risk for high levels of bad cholesterol, boost immunity, and much more.
✓ Chicken soup holds powers that have been acknowledged around the world for centuries as an ancient folk remedy.
✓ However, bone broth is the twenty-first-century superfood that is good for you.
✓ Chicken and turkey heal in a variety of ways—thanks to their low-fat and high-protein content as well as other amazing properties.

Potatoes (Russet/Sweet)

*What I say is that if a man really likes potatoes,
he must be a pretty decent fellow.*
—A. A. MILNE

Chicken soup and bone broth are healing liquids, but potatoes provide superpowers, too. That reminds me of losing loved ones and of superfoods back in my hometown of San Jose. It was a potato kind of day. My dad was in the hospital. One rainy afternoon my sibling and I went on a quest to find my father his go-to comfort food. We stopped at a Wendy's drive-thru. One Classic Chocolate Frosty for dad, and I ordered the Sour Cream and Chive Baked Potato—two superfoods of choice to calm and energize.

Once at our destination, I tried to be the strong daughter. The doctor said, "The prognosis is not good." We were talking weeks before I'd be an orphan. My mind drifted back to the cold chocolate treat and the hot potato. I went back to my father's hospital room and sat on the chair. I can still see the smile on my dad's face when eating the cold, creamy ice cream and feel the calm I reaped from a basic potato. Two comfort superfoods—like daughter and father in sync—shared healing powers that winter day when the sun didn't shine but our spirits were nourished by enjoying life in the moment.

THE HISTORY OF POTATOES

Food historians will tell you the first potato reached Spain in the sixteenth century. Back in 1578, Sir Francis Drake introduced potatoes in his around-the-world adventures. Later, in 1662, it is believed that the British Royal Society sponsored growing potatoes, and by the early 1700s, potatoes were embraced by people in the United States. In grade school, I was taught that sailors on ships ate potatoes to get their vitamin C and fight off the scourge of scurvy. My mom, who was half Irish, used to tell me that the potato was the staple of the Irish diet as she cooked corn beef and cabbage to celebrate Saint Patrick's Day. The bottom line: Potatoes are another versatile superfood, and they deserve credit for all they can do for you and me (thanks to their nutrients).

SUPER NUTRIENTS

Potatoes pack a nutritional punch with a lot of good-for-you nutrients. They are high in vitamins C and B. A large baked potato (these are a challenge to find in the Pacific Northwest and Canada, places where I'm greeted with curly fries or scalloped "taters") contains a mere 220 calories minus the butter and sour cream, which taste delicious but up its calories and fat content. However, topping a baked potato with a dollop of plain Greek yogurt, vegetables, and spices can increase its superfood points.

In graduate school, the student union at San Francisco State University offered a baked potato bar with all the trimmings, which I may have talked about before but deserves to be brought up again. Imagine the toppings, including cheeses, crucifers, chives, mushrooms, and tomatoes. It was a budget-friendly struggling-student's dream come true to eat something hot and nutritious and healthful, too.

Potatoes—both sweet and russet varieties—contain super nutrients. And because they also contain carbohydrates, they may help people calm down and soothe their nerves, as that potato did the last time I spent bonding with my father. Carbohydrates, like potatoes, have a naturally calming effect, which may be due to brain chemistry. According to well-known research done at the Massachusetts Institute of

Technology in Cambridge, eating carbs revs up serotonin, a natural tranquilizer found in the brain, which may help people calm down. But the potato can do much more.

HEALTH BENEFITS OF POTATOES

Russet potatoes: The basic potato that you are familiar with contains almost no fat. That means it's a super source to help you lower the risk of developing heart disease. Also, russet potatoes are a super source of potassium, a great superfood to help control blood pressure. These versatile, budget-friendly potatoes, served baked, as potato skins, or in shepherd's pies, soups, salads, and stews, contain compounds called protease inhibitors that may be cancer fighters, according to medical studies.

Sweet taters: While I adore russet potatoes, sweet potatoes are sweet, too. In the southern United States, folks love their sweet potatoes (whether it's as sweet potato fries or sweet potato pie), and it's not just the super taste they're getting. This potato has a whopping amount of vitamin A, which can enhance your immune system to stave off colds, flu, and even cancer. Medical researchers believe the carotene in them can guard against some types of cancers, perhaps because it can boost white blood cell activity in the body. Also, sweets contain fiber and vitamin C—both touted to help lower the risk of developing cancer. Not to forget the fiber that can help keep your cholesterol numbers in check. And with potassium like russets, these potatoes are good for blood pressure, too. These potatoes are almost fat free and are low in calories, making them diet friendly.

It's confirmed, potatoes deserve a superfood status. If you asked me to make my favorite potato dish, it would probably be a vegetarian shepherd's pie. Instead of dishing out my fail-proof recipe, I decided to dish up a comforting potato soup with superfood ingredients fit for royalty.

Super Immunity-Enhancing Chilled Sweet Potato Soup with Maple-Smoked Chile Sauce

❖ ❖ ❖

This cool winter soup might be just as good warmed up, especially with a drizzle of smoky maple chili sauce on top. The flavors are straight out of a global explorer's cookbook. You have sweet potatoes, which can be traced back to both Africa and prehistoric Polynesia, dried peppers brought up to the colonies by the Spanish conquerors of Mesoamerica, and of course, maple syrup from North America.

1 dried ancho chili
2 dried pasilla chilies
4 dried arbol chilies*
2 tablespoons distilled white vinegar
2½ teaspoons kosher salt, plus more to taste
¼ cup maple syrup (Crown Maple, dark color, robust taste)
¾ cup vegetable oil
4 pounds sweet potatoes (about 4 large), peeled and cut into large chunks

1 teaspoon maple sugar, plus more to taste (Crown Maple)
1 teaspoon freshly ground black pepper, plus more to taste
½ cup plain full-fat Greek yogurt
Up to 5 cups chicken or vegetable broth

The three dried chilies used in this sauce are the most commonly used chilies for preparing classic Mexican mole dishes. Many grocery stores now carry these chilies

*If you don't like heat in your dishes, leave out the chilies.

at the end of the spice aisle, but if you can't find them, go to the best Latin American grocery store you can find and ask for them by name.

Put the dried chilies, vinegar, 1½ teaspoons of the salt, and the maple syrup in a food processor. Process the chilies, drizzling in ½ cup of the oil slowly as you go, until you have a smooth mixture that resembles a home-made barbecue sauce. (Add up to ½ cup water if needed.) Set the sauce aside. (You will have about 1½ cups chili sauce; in a sealable container, it will last up to 1 month in the refrigerator.)

Preheat the oven to 350 degrees F, and line a baking sheet with foil. Combine the sweet potatoes with the remaining ¼ cup vegetable oil, maple sugar, black pepper, and the remaining 1 teaspoon salt in a large bowl and toss to coat the sweet potatoes thoroughly. Spread the sweet potatoes on a baking sheet and bake 25–30 minutes, or until soft and slightly browned on the edges. Let cool.

Place the roasted potatoes in a food processor. Add the yogurt and puree the mixture, adding up to 5 cups broth as necessary, until you have a smooth soup consistency. Season with additional salt, pepper, and maple sugar to taste, then transfer to a sealable container and chill until ready to serve. Serve the soup in bowls and top generously with the chili sauce.

Makes 4 servings.
(Courtesy: Crown Maple and *The Crown Maple Guide to Maple Syrup*)

In the next chapter, get your adventurous garb on because we're going sea diving to discover the healing powers of seaweed. I admit it wasn't and probably isn't my number-one favorite food to eat, even if I was stranded on a tropical island, but sea vegetables are a nutritious superfood worth getting to know up closer.

SUPER-IOR HEALING SUPERFOODS FOR THOUGHT

✓ Russet potatoes may help lower the risk of a variety of diseases—thanks to their vitamins and minerals.

✓ Both russet and sweet potatoes heal in a variety of ways—thanks to their antioxidants and other amazing properties.

✓ Potatoes are low in fat and calories but fill you up, and they are a versatile superfood that often makes a meal when paired with other superfoods—and they should be.

✓ Dieters shouldn't avoid potatoes, but should incorporate them in their diet regime to help lose unwanted pounds.

Seaweed

Potatoes are a basic and ancient superfood that's eaten around the world, but seaweed, also called sea vegetables, is a more exotic power food that blindsided me—twice. The second time I went to Hawaii, I met a dog-loving elderly man on the Big Island. One afternoon when sunbathing was nixed due to gray skies and rain, the local offered me a bag full of dulse chips and a bowl of seaweed soup. I had never eaten sea goo. When my host wasn't looking, I slipped the chips into my bag, tossed the soup on the sand, and buried it like a dog taking care of business. He offered more sea broth in a plastic container, but it didn't make it to my hotel room. I vowed to try it again. But I was feeling like a TV *Fear Factor* contestant challenged to eat a spider, so slurping seaweed soup didn't happen that day—rain or shine.

Ironically, years later, the sea vegetables resurrected and came back to haunt me like a thriller film. I was going to be assigned a book on ocean creatures. One company in Maine sent me a lot of stuff from the sea. After the editorial team decided the timing was not right, I exhaled. The bags of strange-looking sea clumps in all sizes and shapes, stuffed in bags on high shelves in the pantry, were tossed into the trash. Strike two. But I promised myself I'd give the grub from the ocean a go of it one day.

THE HISTORY OF SEAWEED

Like shellfish, seaweed, or sea vegetables, has been on Earth since before biblical times. Not only has it been used as a food source, but also for its medicinal healing powers. Since we have seven seas in the world, there is seaweed in each one. Food historians tell us that Chinese writings note, "There is no swelling that is not relieved by seaweed." There are an infinite number of healing powers attributed to sea vegetables, and they may be due to the plentiful nutrients in each one.

SUPER NUTRIENTS

Seaweed comes in several varieties, and some can be eaten raw in salads and vegetable savory smoothies, others can be cooked and added to soups and casseroles. Any way you discover you like it (remember, it took me a long time), you'll be thrilled to know sea vegetables contain a lot of vitamins and minerals such as iodine, calcium, and iron as well as disease-fighting, immune-boosting antioxidants.

HEALTH BENEFITS OF SEAWEED

Medical doctors, nutritionists, health spa workers, and researchers all agree that seaweed provides healing powers. For starters, since seaweed contains antioxidants, it's not surprising that it may lower the risk of developing cancer. Researchers have found that seaweed not only helps detoxify the body, but it also may protect it from environmental toxins. In fact, some medical experts believe one reason cancer may be less prevalent in Japan than in the United States is because of seaweed being a superfood in the Asian diet.

The superpowers of sea vegetables are no stranger to doctors like

New York–based Fred Pescatore, M.D., M.P.H. He says, "These are a wonderful source of protein for vegans because they contain amino acids and phytonutrients to support good health." He is hardly alone with his observation, even though most sea vegetables used in food—excluding sushi—are not mainstream in the twenty-first century but may, indeed, grow in popularity because of their versatile healing benefits. Here, take a look at some of the most popular sea vegetables, what they are, what they can do, and how to use each one.

Dulse is found in Canadian waters. It is a good source of iron and protein. It is often eaten raw or in soups and salads. Researchers in Oregon claim the seaweed is healthier than kale.

Kelp is rich in iodine and iron.

Nori is the very popular seaweed you may have eaten at a sushi spot. This is the seaweed that wraps around rice rolls.

Wakame is a mix of salty and sweet leaves that are chock-full of bone-boosting calcium and magnesium.

SPIRULINA, THE PERFECT GREEN SUPERFOOD

I recall one medical doctor who touted her love for spirulina—a plant-based protein food—when I asked her about her favorite superfood. At the time, images of the science fiction film *Soylent Green* came to mind. I recalled those little green nutritious wafers (made from recycled people) that were doled out as food during an apocalyptic future scenario that included overpopulation and famine.[1]

These days, I'm more open to this nutrient-dense blue-green algae. It is rich in antioxidants, vitamins, and minerals with a promise to help promote good health and longevity. The doctor called it "clean, good food," and she may be right. It's available in a green powder form—an ideal ingredient for a green smoothie.[2]

Instead of diving into a pool of green superfoods, take it slow by making a spirulina smoothie. I suggest starting with one teaspoon of the green powder and increasing the amount each time you prepare a superfoods smoothie. Try mixing ½ to 1 teaspoon spirulina powder with fresh fruit and green vegetables for a tastier superfood drink: 1/4 cup orange juice, 1/4 cup kale and spinach mix, 1/4 cup apple, 1/2 cup ice, crushed. Blend fruit and vegetables. Add ice. This recipe makes 1 serving.

While my past is rocky when it comes to eating seaweed, I've become a bit more adventurous and so have restaurants, online stores, and even supermarkets where you can find sea vegetables.

Rice Ball (*Onigii*) Nori Sea Vegetable

❖ ❖ ❖

Rice balls are great for backpacking, camping, picnics, breakfast, lunch or dinner, or just a healthy, delicious snack anytime. Yes, I have tried this recipe and it's different but tasty, and teamed with a pot of tea and almond tea cookies it will make you smile, not squirm. I promise.

2 cups precooked short- or medium-grain brown rice
1 umeboshi plum (remove pit) (Eden)
2 sheets sushi nori (Eden)

Lightly moisten your hands with cold water. Take ½ cup cooked rice and form it into a ball, packing it firmly. Poke a hole into the center of the rice ball with your finger and insert ¼ umeboshi plum into the center. Pack the ball again to close the hole, lightly moistening hands if needed.

Fold the nori sheets in half and tear along the fold. Fold in half again and tear on the fold. You should now have eight equal-sized squares of nori about 4 inches by 4 inches—four from each sheet. Lightly moisten your hands, trying not to use much water, and place 1 square of nori on a rice ball, packing until it sticks. Take another square and place it on the rice ball, completely covering the rice ball with nori. Pack gently but firmly to make sure the nori adheres to the rice. Repeat the above steps until you have 4 rice balls completely covered with nori. Eat as you would an apple. Note: Use only leftover short- or medium-grain brown rice to make rice balls. Long grain and basmati rice are not sticky enough to make rice balls.

Makes 4 servings.
(Courtesy: Eden Foods)

SEA SALT

So, I've dished up seaweed, and now here comes sea salt. It's not going to get a superfood title, but it is popular and for good reasons. Have you noticed how many nutrition labels on foods you eat (such as store-bought peanut butter or canned vegetables) list sea salt? Also, I've noticed when viewing Food Network's chefs in competition, they are often reprimanded if salt is left out of a dish, because let's face it, salt adds flavor.

But does sea salt have any nutritional virtues? Some nutritionists believe sea salt is not a bad thing if used in moderation. It does contain some essential nutrients, such as iodine. Also, if you're adding salt to a dish, sea salt seems to be the salt to use in the twenty-first century. If you savor flavorful superfoods (sprinkled with a dash of sea salt) in moderation, that's healthier than overindulging in processed foods with added salt and a superhigh sodium count.

Caveat: Home cooking is a good thing because you can control the salt. When making soup, try using a low-sodium ready-made broth. But as you can see in the following recipe, sea salt gives all the ingredients a burst of flavor.

Super Antiaging Ocean Vegetable Soup

❖ ❖ ❖

1 carton (32 ounces)
   low-sodium organic
   vegetable broth
¼ cup yellow onion
½ cup celery
1 teaspoon thyme
4 Roma tomatoes
Sea salt and freshly
   ground black pep-
   per, to taste

½ cup zucchini,
   chopped
½ cup kale, chopped
2 tablespoons dulse,
   chopped
1½ cups whole-grain
   fettuccine
Parmesan cheese (a
   sprinkle of it for
   each portion)

Pour broth into a large pot. Bring to boil. Add onion, celery, barley, basil, thyme, and tomatoes. Bring to boil again. Add salt and pepper. Then add remaining vegetables, including dulse. Simmer for 15 minutes. In another pot, boil pasta for several minutes until cooked. Drain pasta and add to broth. Simmer for about 10 minutes. Top with cheese.

Makes 4 servings.

Out of the ocean and back on land, follow my lead into the next chapter. I've chosen to focus on a few popular seeds, another one of nature's miracle foods. I may not like sea vegetables, but I love to munch on seeds—ones you know by name, like to eat, and can find at your local supermarket.

SUPER-IOR HEALING SUPERFOODS FOR THOUGHT

✓ Sea vegetables and their multiple healing powers are acknowledged around the world as healing medicines.

✓ Seaweed heals in a variety of ways, from boosting the immune system to lowering your risk of developing cancer—thanks to its antioxidants and other amazing properties.

✓ The wide variety of vegetables from the ocean hold merit for many reasons, especially for vegetarians, and act as versatile substitutes for red meat in salads, soups, and pastas.

Seeds (Pumpkin/Sunflower)

*Don't judge each day by the harvest you reap but
by the seeds that you plant.*
—Robert Louis Stevenson, *Treasure Island*

In between trips to Hawaii and up and down the California coast, I continued to enjoy doing aerobics at the gym and eating a vegetarian diet. One day I was tired of hearing my workout girlfriend's nickname for me—Spindly Arms. At size six, I was a bit frumpy, like the "fat girl," Andy, in *The Devil Wears Prada*. "How could this be?" I asked my gym pal, who was firm and fit. Instead of being a female version of the bullied Piggy in *Lord of the Flies*, I added new superfoods to my diet. I included seeds, including sunflower and pumpkin—the ones I nibbled on to de-stress during college classes in grad school. And I added lifting free weights to my workout regime and stayed clear of the scale.

Within a few months, I was in the locker room and my gal-pal, a former serious body builder, gave me a thumbs-up. While I had gained a few pounds, my biceps, back, thighs, and legs showed definition. I shouted, "I have muscles!" And big credit goes to those little protein-rich seeds (along with eggs and poultry). But note, if you stop eating protein-rich superfoods and pumping iron, you may regress to a Casper the Friendly Ghost–type of body.

THE HISTORY OF SEEDS

Seeds go way, way back to the Paleolithic era, when gatherers would forage for nuts and seeds, which were part of their natural diet. There are a variety of types of edible seeds, including fennel and caraway, but in the modern day, the classic pumpkin seeds and sunflower seeds are favorites, and not to forget super watermelon seeds (once considered a pesky black seed in a slice of juicy watermelon).

SUPER NUTRIENTS

Two seeds I favor are pumpkin and sunflower (not to forget protein-rich sesame seeds) because they taste super and have super nutritional value, too. True, white-colored pumpkin seeds in the shells and sunflower seeds (including the shells) are high in sodium, some calories, and fat. But eating seeds like these in moderation provides superfood perks that are worth you incorporating them into your diet.

Sunflower seeds contain vitamin E and compounds called protease inhibitors, which may help as cancer-fighting superfoods. But you want to eat seeds in moderation as a satisfying nutritional snack (also the crunching helps lower stress) or sprinkled in cereals, salads, stir-frys, and both fruit and vegetable smoothies.

EDIBLE SUPERFOOD SEEDS

There are a variety of good-for-you seeds, and once you start consuming one type, don't be surprised if you enjoy others. Here's a quick glance at some of the most popular seeds available at supermarkets, health food stores, and online stores.

HEALTH BENEFITS OF SEEDS

The fat content in pumpkin and sunflower seeds is mostly the unsaturated kind; this is the good fat to help lower the risk of developing heart disease. Both pumpkin seeds and sunflower seeds are rich in dietary fiber and minerals—also heart-healthy for keeping your cholesterol levels in check.

Seed	Nutrients	Taste, Form, and Uses
Chia	7 grams protein, 200 calories, 18 grams fat, vita-, min E, omega-3 fatty acids	Nutty flavor; raw; cereal, Greek yogurt
Flax	8 grams protein, 224 calo-, ries, 18 grams fat, omega-3 fatty acids	Nutty flavor; whole or ground; salads, smoothies, Greek yogurt
Pumpkin	8 grams protein, 224 calories, 13 grams fat	Sweet; baking toppings, salads, snacks
Sesame	6 grams protein, 208 calories, 18 grams fat, antioxidants	Small, crunchy; candy, cookies
Sunflower	7 grams protein, 204 calories, vitamins B and E, 18 grams fat	Crunchy; raw, shelled; salads, snacking
Watermelon	312 calories, manganese, magnesium, zinc, low in fat and sodium	Soft and chewy; snacking

(Sources: Manufacturer's products; USDA)

You do not want to eat cups of seeds (although if you're not mindful, it's easy to do) if you want to keep your weight in check. Also, salted sunflower seeds and pumpkin seeds (super high in sodium) can raise your blood pressure. So, the key is moderation for the health perks, and seeds can do a body good. (See Chapter 25, "Home Remedies from Your Kitchen," for more on the health benefits of pumpkin seeds for men.)

Super Revitalizing Peanut Butter and Jam Thumbprint Cookies

❖ ❖ ❖

My mom baked large, old-fashioned peanut butter cookies, the kind with a crisscross imprint on top. I created a smaller thumbprint peanut butter cookie filled with superfood nut butter, inspired by the good old days when peanut butter got me through those fancy meals that weren't my fancy when my mother enjoyed the thrill of making foods from different cultures.

2½ cups whole-wheat flour (King Arthur)

1½ teaspoons baking soda

1½ teaspoons baking powder

Dash of sea salt

½ cup all-natural peanut butter

½ cup all-natural almond or cashew butter

⅓ cup European-style unsalted butter

¼ cup light-brown sugar

¼ cup white granulated sugar

1 organic brown egg

1 teaspoon pure vanilla extract

½ cup peanuts, chopped

½ cup organic berry jam, (O Organics)

½ cup raw pumpkin or sunflower seeds

Preheat oven to 400 degrees F. In a bowl, combine flour, baking soda, baking powder, and salt. Add soft butters, sugars, and egg, and cream them. Mix in vanilla. Fold in peanuts. Form cookie dough into a roll and wrap in parchment paper. Chill for at least an hour. Slice dough into ¼-inch slices, roll into balls, and place on ungreased cookie sheet. Use your thumb to make an imprint to place jam. Bake for about 10 minutes. Once out of the oven, place jam on each cookie. Sprinkle with seeds.

Makes approximately 3 dozen cookies.

In the next pages, we're going to dive back into the deep blue sea. This time, though, we're getting reintroduced to shellfish. While seaweed is probably the most unusual functional food I dish up, shellfish can titillate taste buds for most people (if they are not allergic). Move over salmon (fatty fish is a popular and touted superfood), the spotlight is now on the forgotten fish of the ocean.

SUPER-IOR HEALING SUPERFOOD FOR THOUGHT

✓ Seeds may help lower the risk of developing cancers, reduce levels of bad cholesterol, boost immunity, and much more.

✓ Both sunflower and pumpkin seeds heal in a variety of ways— thanks to their antioxidants and other amazing properties.

✓ Seeds provide a lot of essential nutrients, including plant-based proteins.

✓ All types of seeds are extremely versatile since they can be used for health, taste, and texture in salads, smoothies, breads, and cereals—making any diet more healthful.

Shellfish

He was a bold man that first ate an oyster.
—JONATHAN SWIFT, *Gulliver's Travels*

My memories of the Hawaiian Islands (despite my angst about edible sea monsters) are delightful, but shellfish are a different ocean tale in my book (pun intended). On the Big Island, after scanning the fish plates on the hotel restaurant menu, my frugal mate didn't want to dine on a fish dinner; we ended up at his favorite place, McDonald's. He ordered a hamburger; I nibbled on French fries while planning a homemade shellfish dinner for one. In my mind, on that night in Hawaii while recalling shellfish dishes on the food menu, my affair with fish grew into a Hemingway-like romantic passage from *A Moveable Feast* about "oysters with their strong taste of the sea" that helped me be rid of the "empty feeling and began to be happy."

On my own again, back on the mainland, I revisited Cannery Row, a place I love, and revisited a restaurant in Monterey, California, overlooking the Pacific Ocean. For old time's sake, I ordered cioppino, an Italian-American fisherman's stew, to get my refill of shellfish—lobster, shrimp, clams, and oysters. "It's time," like the character Felipe (Javier Bardem) says in the film *Eat Pray Love* film before making love. And now it's time I introduce my desire for crustaceans and mollusks—"new" superfoods that warrant more love.

THE HISTORY OF SHELLFISH

Shellfish are nothing new. Crabs and shrimp have been swimming in the sea around the globe since the beginning of time. From the Stone Age days on into century after century, the ocean around the globe has been a food source for all cultures—and shellfish have been well received from ancient days to the present day—and for good reason.

Of course, shellfish have been gathered and dished up at waterfront restaurants in coastal regions, which I've experienced, from San Francisco to Seattle, New Orleans to South Carolina, and up north to Maine. Not only are shellfish a historical wonder eaten by people in the United States and around the world, they're also nutritious. Also important is consuming sustainable shellfish. Simply put, these are fish caught in ways that include the continuation of harvested varieties and the well-being of seafood-dependent communities.

SUPER NUTRIENTS

The good diet news about shellfish from the deep sea is that they are diet friendly because overall they are not high in calories; a ½-cup serving of fresh crab is 105 calories, whereas meat contains more calories. They are a dieter's friend because they are low in saturated fat and calories.

In favor of shellfish, type by type, they contain some essential minerals, including calcium and protein. However, shellfish do have the reputation of being high in cholesterol and sodium, so they must be eaten and savored in moderation, and then you can reap super merits worth every bite, especially when they are paired with other superfoods, such as leafy greens, lemon juice, tomatoes, and whole grains.

TYPES OF SHELLFISH

The shellfish type called crustaceans includes crab, lobster, and shrimp—three of my favorite for a long time. Crab louie or shrimp louie and a decadent lobster tail dipped in butter come to mind when I go back to some memorable dishes I've enjoyed at restaurants at

Fisherman's Wharf in San Francisco, on the Bay Area peninsula, and Avalon on Catalina Island.

Shrimp: A 3-ounce serving has 17 grams of protein, nine amino acids, and some minerals such as selenium; this serving contains almost half of the recommended dietary allowance for this cancer-fighting nutrient. Also, a serving of shrimp contains about one-third of the recommended dietary allowance for vitamin D (key for seniors and people who do not get enough sunshine).

Crab: Fresh crab—not the canned variety—is delicious and like shrimp does have nutritional perks. Eating softshell crabs takes work, but its fun and they are delicious. Crab is low in calories, and in a salad like a crab louie can be a diet-friendly meal.

Lobster: Not unlike shrimp, lobster has a whopping 19 grams of protein and nine amino acids. It's a rich and pricey shellfish, but on occasion is worth the splurge. Small amounts included in a pasta dish or soup are delicious as well as nutritious. But if you view the film *Julie & Julia*, cover your eyes and ears when you hear the words "Lobster killer, lobster killer."

Welcome to mollusks, the other group of shellfish, including clams, oysters, and scallops. These fish, not unlike crustaceans, are rich in proteins, low in fat, and super rich in essential nutrients, like zinc.

Clams: A small, 3-ounce serving of this shellfish provides 700 percent of the recommended dietary allowance for vitamin B_{12}, which helps with brain health and your nervous system, and more than half of the recommended dietary allowance for iron, which is necessary to provide energy and stave off anemia. (Iron is especially important for women of all ages, but probably more important during the child-bearing years and if a woman is a vegetarian.)

Oysters: These shellfish are nature's gift from the ocean. Eight ounces of oysters contain 100 percent of the recommended dietary allowance of zinc, which helps power up the immune system and is important for people of all ages and both genders.

Scallops: They are a favorite superfood fish of mine since I was a kid. My mom served breaded scallops paired with fish sticks. These round gems provide about 80 percent of the recommended dietary allowance of protein, making them a super source if you're a part-time vegan/vegetarian, like I am and continue to be.

CATCHING A NUTRITIOUS SEAFOOD

All of these shellfish are rich in protein and omega-3 fatty acids. They are good for weight loss and getting essential nutrients, but more is less to avoid getting too much cholesterol and sodium.

Shellfish (½ cup)	Calories	Some Key Super Nutrients
Clams	86	Vitamin B_{12}, vitamin C, iron, niacin, potassium, phosphorus, zinc
Crab	105	Vitamin C, vitamin B_{12}, copper, folate, magnesium, selenium, zinc
Lobster	108	Vitamin B_{12}, copper, phosphorus, potassium, selenium, zinc
Shrimp	90	Vitamin B_{12}, phosphorus, selenium, zinc
Oysters	103	Vitamin B_{12}, vitamin C, copper, iron, magnesium, niacin, selenium, zinc
Scallops	127	Vitamin B_{12}, calcium, copper, iron, phosphorus, potassium, selenium

HEALTH BENEFITS OF SHELLFISH

Shellfish (all types) are high-protein, low-calorie superfoods that provide a variety of health virtues (unless you are allergic to them!). Wild salmon is often the number-one fish on superfood lists, but shellfish deserve a thumbs-up, too.

Since shellfish—all types—are lower in calories than meat such as a cut of steak, and lower in fat, this makes them a healthier choice of protein, which we need from head to toe (brain health to stronger nails and hair). Also, the extra calories in meat come from fat, whereas a serving of scallops has a mere 5 grams of fat; beef has up to 20 grams of artery-clogging fat—not good news for cholesterol and heart disease.

And those little shrimp you love to eat provide a big carotenoid known for its healthful antioxidant action, which research shows may help lower the risk of developing cancer and heart disease. Also, lobster passes up shrimp for its content of the cancer-fighting mineral selenium, with more than 50 percent of the recommended dietary allowance in just the 3 ounces you can get in a tasty shrimp cocktail.

Interestingly, both shrimp and lobster have been shunned because of their reputation of high dietary cholesterol. Past research findings have shown these shellfish can actually raise "good" HDL cholesterol and lower triglycerides (a risk for heart disease).

The heart-healthy Oldways Mediterranean diet does include shellfish (in moderation). Keep in mind, members of coastal cultures, such as native Hawaiians and Eskimos in Alaska, who eat fish have lower disease rates than people who consume too much meat. Caveat: It's important, too, however, to know the source of your fresh shellfish and to cook and store it properly for your health's sake and to avoid bacteria.

Super Protein-Boosting Seafood Gumbo

❖ ❖ ❖

I adore a fish soup, where you wear a bib, crack fresh shellfish, and eat it with French bread. But I chose this recipe because the creator is a seasoned cook and knows how to prepare seafood with finesse. Fish is an excellent way to get protein, an essential nutrient for your muscles, bones, and body.

4 tablespoons flour
4 tablespoons olive oil
 (Marsala olive oil)
1 onion, chopped (or scallion)
1 cup celery, chopped
1 bell pepper, chopped
1 cup okra, fresh or
 frozen, chopped into
 1-inch pieces
4 garlic cloves (or to
 taste)
2 zucchini, diced
2 cups fresh tomatoes,
 chopped
2 tablespoons tomato
 paste
2 bay leaves
Cayenne, to taste
1 tablespoon
 Worcestershire sauce
1 cup white wine
1 cup water or broth
½ pound shrimp, medium,
 cleaned
½ pound crab meat,
 picked over
½ pound white fish fillets
 (your choice), cut into
 about 1-inch cubes
2 cups oysters or crayfish
 tails
½ cup basil, chopped (or
 parsley)
Sea salt and pepper to
 taste

In large heavy Dutch oven (a large, heavy pan with a lid that can be used on a stove top or in the oven), over low heat, stir flour and oil together until smooth. Cook, stirring often, until mixture turns golden brown, about 10 minutes. Add onion, celery, peppers, okra, and garlic, cook until tender. Add zucchini, tomatoes, tomato paste, bay leaves, cayenne, and Worcestershire sauce, cook about 20 minutes. Add wine and water, bring to a boil, lower heat. Add seafood and basil, simmer until shrimp are pink, 5–8 minutes, and when fillets flake easily with a fork. Add basil. Remove bay leaves before serving. Sprinkle salt and pepper to taste. Serve with cooked rice or couscous.

Makes 6 servings.
(Courtesy: Gemma Sanita Sciabica, from *Cooking with California Olive Oil: Popular Recipes*)

Now that I've put shellfish on the table, it's time to bring in another superfood—one that pairs well with shellfish from the sea. Let's take a look at tomatoes, big and small, chopped, sliced, diced, raw, and cooked, and find out what's in those red gems that you love in salads, soups, pastas, and more.

SUPER-IOR HEALING SUPERFOODS FOR THOUGHT

✓ Shellfish may help lower the risk of developing cancers, reduce levels of bad cholesterol, boost immunity, and much more.

✓ Shellfish heal in a variety of ways—thanks to their antioxidants and other amazing vitamins and minerals.

✓ From crabs to oysters, shellfish and their versatility belong in every diet.

✓ Shellfish can be budget friendly if purchased when in season, frozen, or canned.

✓ Shellfish, eaten in moderation, can be an ideal protein-rich addition to a heart-healthy lifestyle.

CHAPTER

19

Tomatoes

Of the tomato or love apple,
I know very little.
—WILLIAM ANDRUS ALCOTT, *The Young House-Keeper*

Like shellfish, tomatoes have a place in my heart and diet. Months after the breakup with the fast-food man, I met a body builder at the gym. Our bond was carbs. After working out, my new friend asked, "Do you have any pasta?" I shook my head no so we stopped at the store. He picked up a bottle of generic vegetable oil, one jar of no-name marinara sauce, and refined white pasta. I was thrilled my friend offered to create a pasta plate. (I hid the fact that I knew how to cook.) But thanks to my beloved Brittany spaniel's allergy to the anticanine cook, there wasn't a *Lady and the Tramp* human sequel of pulling each other into a kiss when slurping up the same noodle from the plate of spaghetti.

The next day, I brought home a bag filled with tomatoes—off the vine from a neighbor. I cooked up homemade tomato sauce with superfoods, including cheeses, extra-virgin olive oil, and whole-grain pasta for lasagna. The chunks of juicy tomatoes with notes of fresh herbs were lovely, and I shared a piece of pasta with my loyal dog, who appreciated my cooking skills, sensed I was content (once again) with my single status, and was delighted with my entrée that was chock-full of real tomatoes.

THE HISTORY OF TOMATOES

Initially, the bright red, juicy tomato was recognized by 500 B.C. and grown in Mexico. It was sacred to the Pueblo people, who believed that those who watched others eat tomato seeds were blessed with being able to forecast the future. The tomato, which is a summer fruit, can be grown and shipped from around the world, so it is available year-round.

SUPER NUTRIENTS

Tomatoes—all varieties, big and small—are low in calories and fat. A whole cup of chopped tomatoes boasts fewer than 50 calories and contains potassium, vitamin C, vitamin A, B-complex vitamins, potassium, and phosphorus.

When I traveled to Victoria, British Columbia, and ordered a salad for an afternoon snack, I met my first heirloom tomato. Darker in color than a Roma variety (my longtime tomato of choice for salads, sauces and soups), it was sweet and was an instant pleasant taste and memory that I took home and used in many tomato recipes, from soups to salads and even smoothies. Sun-dried tomatoes aren't my cup of tea, and cherry tomatoes are fun for appetizers.

But it's vine-ripened tomatoes—the popular "go-to slicers"—that I know from being a kid and growing up in a semifarming region. As a starving student (peanut butter sandwiches and potatoes were my constant friends), every day I passed by a vegetable field run by local farmers near my apartment in San Jose. One day at dusk, I snuck under an opening in the barbed wire fence. I collected vine-ripened tomatoes and put them in my knapsack. The pilfered tomatoes were juicy and delicious, making hoagie sandwiches worth the robbery. And once you savor the real tomato, purchasing other types just isn't the same decadent experience.

HEALTH BENEFITS OF TOMATOES

It's no shocker that this low-fat, low-calorie, and nutrient-plentiful fruit (the tomato is not a vegetable) is a heart-healthy food and may lower the risks of developing heart disease and cancer. Not unlike potatoes, tomatoes are a versatile superfood and are used in appetizers, salads, soups, entrees, and even smoothies.

Tomatoes also contain the superantioxidant lycopene (as noted in chapter 12, the chapter on pizza). One tomato provides a whopping amount of cancer-fighting of lycopene and vitamin C. Stacks of research show that the antioxident lycopene (found in fresh tomatoes, like those used in the recipe below, tomato paste, and tomato sauce) not only may lower the risk of developing many types of cancer, it may also help lower the risk of heart disease and lower the levels of "bad" cholesterol.

Super Comforting End-of-Season Fried Green Tomatoes

The movie *Fried Green Tomatoes* introduced me to this tomato dish, which I've grown to love. As a dish for a hot summer night or a warm spring afternoon snack, these tomatoes are delicious and will wow your family, friends, or simply you. Enjoy each and every crispy, juicy bite.

1 egg, beaten
4 green tomatoes with
   pink blush, sliced
   ¼-inch thick
1 cup cornmeal
4 cloves garlic, or to taste,
   minced

2 tablespoons rosemary,
   minced, or basil
⅓ cup Marsala extra-virgin
   olive oil (Sciabica's)
Salt and pepper, to
   taste

In pie plate, beat egg slightly. In another pie plate, mix cornmeal, garlic, and rosemary or basil. Dip tomato slices in beaten egg on both sides, then dredge in cornmeal. Cook in skillet with olive oil until tender and crisp on the outside. Season with salt and pepper. (Author's note: I used ½ cup panko and ½ cup cornmeal for a crunchy texture.)

(Courtesy: Gemma Sanita Sciabica, from *Cooking with California Olive Oil: Recipes for the Heart from the Heart*)

As you near the end of my chosen top 20 superfoods, water is a top pick. You may take water for granted, but when you discover all the reasons why mankind needs it, you may rethink this pick and understand why it made the short list.

SUPER-IOR HEALING SUPERFOODS FOR THOUGHT

✓ Tomatoes—all varieties and there are a lot—may help lower the risk of developing cancers, boost immunity, and much more.
✓ All types of tomatoes and their powers are acknowledged around the world as healing medicines.
✓ Tomatoes, not unlike other lycopene-rich cancer-fighting foods (such as orange and red fruits and vegetables) have amazing properties to boost your immune system—thanks to their antioxidants.
✓ The almighty tomato is rich in a lot of essential nutrients, which earns it superstar status as a garden-fresh superfood.
✓ Tomatoes are available in different ways in addition to fresh ones, such as tomato paste, canned tomatoes, and tomato juice, which all provide healing powers.

Water (Watermelon) and . . .

High and fine literature is wine, and mine is only
water; but everyone likes water.
—MARK TWAIN

Life in the mountains has fueled my love of water (from the view of
the lake to swimming at resort pools), and during a trip to Victoria,
British Columbia, water played a role, too. It wasn't the fresh melon
chunks at the breakfast buffet that wowed me, though, or the early
morning swim and hot tub—although they are lovely; after all, drinking water and physical activity are part of a healthy diet (whatever type
you follow) and lifestyle.

One of my goals was to take a boat tour on the Gorge (a once popular water boat hub that flows into the Inner Harbour and the open
Pacific Ocean). I sipped bottled water to stay hydrated during the
45-minute event while enjoying the smooth water and the locals
kayaking and swimming.

After the boat ride (which spawned images of when I went to Catalina Island via boat and a sailboat trip in San Francisco Bay), I found a
smoothie stand, an attraction for tourists. Since I survived the water

adventure (there was no rogue wave or rough water), I ordered a cantaloupe smoothie. I was not formerly a melon lover (except for watermelon in the summertime), so it was a wake-up call that water-rich melons are a superfruit worth including in the list of superfoods.

Years ago, I was reminded by one doctor about the importance of water; the human body is made up of 50 to 70 percent of the liquid, and H_2O is an essential superfood. As a fan of sci-fi films, I've watched in horror when our hero or heroine doesn't have water because the drama soars as we wait for them to get gulps of water to survive. *Castaway* and *Thirst*—both movies showed the grave need for water to stay alive.[1]

Not to forget real-life stories, from bad water in our own country to lack of water around the world. Do you remember Erin Brockovich's mission to link disease to bad water tied to dumping toxic waste into the groundwater and the current water crisis in Flint, Michigan, due to drinking water from a polluted river? Both incidents spawned films based on good water gone bad, which makes you wonder if the tap water you're drinking is safe. Also, when natural disasters hit, one of the first things people are advised to do is stock up on water. So why? Why in the world is water so important, anyhow?

THE HISTORY OF WATER

Water goes back to the beginning of time. No, not bottled or filtered water, but people in the caveman era through biblical times and on into century after century would get their fresh water from lakes and rivers. Throughout history, getting untainted water was of paramount importance, as people needed to stay clear of water that needed treatment to get rid of pollutants.

Writings from ancient Greece show that boiling and filtering water through charcoal were used to purify it, along with exposing water to sunlight and straining it. Egyptians used alum to remove particles by 1500 B.C., and water continued to be filtered for healthful drinking through the medieval era. The Romans were on top of getting clean water using their aqueducts. London's New River was constructed in the early seventeenth century as a means of bringing clean water from outside the city.[2]

SUPER NUTRIENTS

Pure water is good, and its nutrients are super great. Water has zero calories, fat, sodium, and sugar—a dieter's dream. Also, drinking healthy water without fat or cholesterol can help lower your risk of developing heart disease and obesity, a scourge for both men and women.

Since healthy drinking water keeps the body functioning properly, it is a fact that it is essential for good nutrition and basic survival. You can live without food much longer than you can without water.

HEALTH BENEFITS OF WATER

Water is one doctor's favorite superfood. Meet Dr. Kevin D. Jenkins, D.C., a chiropractor in Las Vegas, Nevada. "Without water I feel like an old man," he told me when I interviewed him for my book *Doctors' Orders*. Since our body is made up of water (which varies on age and size), it makes sense. We need water to replenish our cells; it keeps you hydrated, energized, "regular," and much more.

"I wake up in the morning and drink a quart of water the first thing," adds Dr. Jenkins. "I feel better when I do that. I do martial arts, and when I don't get enough water the next morning I feel arthritic because my body has not been able to get the toxins out." And note, the average person should drink a minimum of seven to eight 8-ounce glasses per day.[3]

But note, drinking unhealthy water containing impurities, like after a natural disaster, can be a life-threatening situation. It is advised to store one gallon of water per person for seven days in case of an emergency situation.

WATER AND WEIGHT LOSS

When I was in my late teens and a know-it-all, I stayed lean by crash dieting, working out in a gym with free weights, and swimming. I thought by not drinking water, I would keep my tummy flat, but then I'd get thirsty and drink a lot and gain the water weight right back. It didn't cross my mind that dehydration was a possibility. After all, I was young and invincible, right? Wrong.

Water is a dieter's best friend. Health professor Ruopeng An, Ph.D., of the University of Illinois and other researchers discovered that by upping your water consumption by one to three cups per day, you may eat from 68 to 2,015 fewer calories per day. The study, published in the *Journal of Human Nutrition and Dietetics*, included not only lab rats but nearly twenty thousand people who not only experienced a cut in calories, but also ate less fat, sugar, sodium, and cholesterol. The findings: fewer calories, more weight loss.[4]

These days, older and wiser, I am always sipping water—not just tea. It takes the place of mindless eating, and I, like the people in the study, do not overindulge in processed foods because I'm not hungry. I'm satisfied. Caveat: If you ditch sugary or diet sodas and replace them with water and drink seven to eight 8-ounce glasses per day for 30 days, I promise you that you will not go back to the no-water days. Drinking water and enjoying its benefits will be a habit and a healthy one.

Bottled or Tap Water?

The controversy about tap water versus bottled or filtered water continues. Dr. Jenkins prefers mountain spring water because too many of the other types have been filtered or have chemical additives that may cause their own host of problems. For years, I've been drinking bottled water (it is advised to use glass containers instead of plastic, which may contain contaminants) because of the threat of the groundwater and its chemicals in the mountains. We used to receive letters about arsenic in the groundwater. Then, water companies discussed contaminated wells in South Lake Tahoe.[5]

Making the choice to drink tap or bottled water also depends on where you live or visit when traveling. My younger brother, for instance, went to Cabo, Mexico. He was diligent about not drinking any tap water. However, he did brush his teeth and drank beverages with ice cubes. The last night of the trip, it happened. He spent hours in the bathroom. So, was the water in a foreign country to blame? The answer will never be known, but I know when traveling bottled water is my choice.

WATER-FILLED WATERMELON

Watermelons, honeydew melons, and cantaloupes all have something in common. These are water-dense superfruits. Drinking water is important, but you can get water in other superfoods, too—including melons.

As a youngster, I loved eating a slice of cold watermelon after swimming next door in the hot summertime, but I passed on cantaloupe for breakfast. (I didn't like its squishy texture because it reminded me of beans.) And honeydew balls were pretty and fun to play with in a bowl, but not something my palate preferred. What did I know? I was just a kid.

Let's talk watermelon. Since it's a potassium-rich superfruit, it can help fight bloat. Yes, it can get rid of water retention and flatten the belly. Watermelon acts as a natural diuretic, which can help lessen the feel and look of belly bloat.

Potassium works on the body to counteract sodium—a culprit that can cause you to retain water and feel pudgy in the tummy. But eating a slice of watermelon (it is 90 percent water) can help you to attain a flatter stomach so you'll feel more comfortable in your favorite jeans or dress. A creative salad with melon balls is superfoods at their best.

Melon Bowl Salad with Fruit-Flavored Water

❖ ❖ ❖

After my trip to Victoria, British Columbia, images of the hotel's dinner appetizers were on my mind. While I adopted the cheese plate, why not add fresh melon to my diet repertoire, right? But when I saw those adorable miniwatermelons at the supermarket, things changed.

I always wanted to make one of those attractive, eye-catching melon bowl salads, artfully designed with an assortment of colorful melon balls—and I did just that, sort of. This recipe is inspired by my trip to Victoria and fond memories of flying in the plane and seeing the dark blue water while landing on the island.

1 seedless miniwatermelon or cantaloupe

1½ cups assorted melon, balls or cubes

1 cup mixed fruit (apples, grapes)

2 tablespoons honey

1 teaspoon fresh lemon juice

Cinnamon, to taste

½ cup Greek yogurt (Greek Gods Yogurt)

Mint leaves for garnish

Using a sharp knife, slice a thick slice from bottom of melon to make a flat base so melon will lie nicely on a dish or bowl. Slice melon in half. Scoop out melon to leave shell intact. Slice the melon into square chunks or use a melon ball scoop and scoop out balls. Place melon chunks in a bowl. Add fruit. Mix in honey, lemon, and cinnamon. Cover and chill in refrigerator. Top with a scoop of vanilla Greek yogurt. Garnish with fresh mint leaves.

Serves 2.

Super Refreshing and Calming Fruit-Flavored Water

Store-bought flavored waters, like coconut water, are popular. I have tried some of the infused flavorful waters available on the market, but when I noted additives on the nutrition label, it was back to nature and making fruit-flavored water myself.

16 ounces water, bottled or filtered
2 slices each orange and lemon or lime
Fresh mint leaves for garnish

In a tall glass, pour water, and place citrus in it. Top with mint.

Makes 2 servings.

Now that you've got the scoop on water (and water-rich superfruit) for your health's sake—and survival—it's time to bring onboard other beverages. Other types of beverages can provide extra healthy nutrients, as you'll find out in the next chapter.

SUPER-IOR HEALING SUPERFOODS FOR THOUGHT

✓ Superfood water may help lower the risk of dehydration and heart disease, and up the odds of keeping you alive.

✓ Clean, pure water and its powers are acknowledged around the world as a healing medicine and vital for good health.

✓ Water, including tea and watermelon, heals in many ways—thanks to its super-antioxidants, vitamins, and minerals.

... Other Healthy Beverages

Wine is bottled poetry.
—ROBERT LOUIS STEVENSON

I've doled out water love from my escapades in Victoria, British Columbia, but there was another beverage incident during that trip to Canada that I'd like to share with you, too. When waiting for my flight to the island at Seattle-Tacoma International Airport, I was sleep deprived due to leaving home at 2:30 A.M. At 3:30 P.M., it hit me. I befriended a fellow baby boomer traveler. The New Yorker (who resembled the intellectual celebrity chef Alton Brown) told me he was on his way to a meditation retreat in Victoria. I looked at him and said, "I need coffee. I want to feel normal." He responded, "You'll regret it. Go with the jet lag; you'll be fine tomorrow." I wondered why he traveled so far to chill when he could have gotten "spa'd" in upstate New York. But I fled Tahoe tourists during the Fourth of July to find a sense of calm, so, maybe he was right.

Flying in a CRJ700 (a small aircraft) was a phobia of mine, so caffeine in a cup of joe wasn't the cure. At the café, I bought a bottled water and an orange juice. I mixed the two drinks to avoid the sugar rush of the OJ. (It didn't look pretty like the fruit-infused water containers at health spas, but it had less sugar than ready-made juice drinks.) And I did get a boost of immune-boosting vitamin C (to stave off getting sick from on-the-road germs). I felt awake and balanced on the plane. (Okay. I give credit to some juice sugar and no rough air.) Caveat: While I was relaxed, the elderly Australian woman sitting next to me could have benefited from my DIY beverage, I thought, as I watched her adjust a headset. (It was a calming nature tape, she whispered to me.) She placed an eye mask over her eyes. She apologized and whispered to me, "I'm a nervous flier." I smiled, ascending into the air while anticipating the breathtaking scenery of the island. No jitters. It had to be the water–orange juice high, and I was calm and centered.

THE HISTORY OF JUICE

Since biblical times, health-conscious people have used juice fasting for its body-detoxing benefits. In the 1900s, juicing was a growing trend. There is a Japanese vegetable juice drink made from kale or barley grass. It was created in 1943 by Dr. Nero Endo, who experimented with vegetable juices.[1]

In the sixties and seventies, juicing (especially fruit juice) was a trend. Later on, green drinks and juicing became popular in the eighties. And I jumped on the juice-fast bandwagon. Read on to find out if the juice diet really works.

The Juice-Detox Fast

In the Santa Cruz Mountains, on Highway 9, at a small store, I purchased a few types of juice (apple, orange, and grape) so I wouldn't get bored. I wasn't hungry. Throughout the day, I drank water and fruit juice drinks. On the second day I did experience a lot of down time in the bathroom. I felt it was a good thing; my body was detoxing itself. I felt more energized. I had images of food, such as hamburgers and French fries, but I didn't cave. After day two, I was craving clean foods in my mind, but I still wasn't hungry. When I stepped onto the scale, I was amazed. I had dumped five pounds. It was a super jump-start diet.

SUPER NUTRIENTS

The nutrients in fruit juices should be the same as the vitamins and minerals you get from the vegetables and fruits. Using the whole fruit—including the skin, too—is fine for some fruits (obviously not a banana). But note, use organic produce for health's sake.

Juicing and its nutritional perks are controversial, like umpteen other health and diet topics. Some health experts will tell you that you lose dietary fiber, while others will tell you it's good to give your body a rest from fiber. The majority of health gurus will tell you—and I agree—that the added sugars in store-bought juices (worse if they are not 100 percent juice) are not healthy and make them less than a superfood. So whole fruit is best—juiced or not.

HEALTH BENEFITS OF JUICE

Still, in the twenty-first century, both health-conscious spa-goers and health-food-store fans do gravitate to green drinks, but they aren't for the unsophisticated palate. Adding a few greens in a vegetable or fruit juice drink may be one way to keep the trend going in the coming decades by appealing to a mainstream fan base.

The healing powers of juice are infinite, depending on what source you use. Both superfruits and supervegetables—solo or paired—contain vitamins and mineral as well as antioxidants that can help you keep your weight in check and lower your risk of developing heart disease and cancer. Medical doctors and nutritionists in the twenty-first century will tell you fresh fruit and vegetable juices can flush toxins from your body. Juice fasting for a short span of time (a few days is ideal) is like taking your body on a minivacation. You'll likely feel rejuvenated.

WHAT ABOUT RED WINE?

More than once people have said to me (a self-professed type-A individual who has difficulty relaxing), "You should start drinking red wine." But due to my genes, I've chosen to stay clear of alcohol. Still, that doesn't mean I don't know about the healing powers of red wine, and I have pondered the question of what if I did indulge in a glass of the red stuff, which is an idea still on the table.

When I wrote the book *The Healing Powers of Vinegar*, the topic of red wine and its link to red wine vinegar was introduced to me. It was a brilliant concept, and I dug into it like a dog searching for its bone. So, as I delved into research and interviewed wine experts, I was reminded that wine comes from healthful grapes, found in regions like Central California, with its warm and humid Mediterranean climate. And we know grapes, whether fresh, as natural juice, or fermented as wine, are a super source of flavonoids—powerful phenolic compounds that act to protect your body from disease.

As I've noted earlier, flavonoids are super disease fighters that may help lower the risk of developing allergies, colds, flu, inflammation, and even heart disease and cancer. Other powerful compounds in grapes include a myriad of antioxidants, including proanthocyanidin, quercetin, and resveratrol, which may have anticancer properties and guard against heart disease.[2]

In the late twentieth century, resveratrol was a buzzword. Simply put, this natural compound in grapes may play a role in producing healthy cholesterol levels, zapping unhealthy fats in the bloods, and even preventing blood clotting in arteries narrowed by years of eating a high-fat diet. Since heart disease is still the number-one killer in both men and women, resveratrol seems like a good thing to add to a heart healthy diet. And there's more.

While red wine contains resveratrol, so does grape juice. I interviewed one researcher who told me that grapes and anything made from grapes that includes the grape skin contains resveratrol. Research continues to show that resveratrol not only does help lower levels of bad cholesterol, it may also reduce the risk of developing cancer. So, if you, like me, don't drink alcohol, perhaps we should add grape juice to our diet. Actually, I did purchase organic grape juice, and it sits in my refrigerator.

For weeks, it was on my to-do list to create a grape juice smoothie, and I finally did it one warm, winter day. Here is the easy recipe: ½ cup grape juice, ½ cup orange juice, ¼ cup plain Greek yogurt, ¼ cup red grapes, ¼ cup apples, ¼ cup ice cubes. Blend until thick and creamy. And this is how to get your resveratrol and drink it, too.

Yes, drinking organic red wine or eating grapes and drinking grape juice (without pesticides or added sugar) can healthy-up a diet, but no it's not a magic bullet to good health. Some scientists, as I noted before, believe attaching superfood labels to superfruits like grapes or grape juice is a marketing tool, but I disagree. Saying these foods are heart-healthy raises awareness and helps us to eat, drink, and be merry, and it may be helpful in adding quality years to our lifespans.

Meanwhile, my memories of traveling to Napa's olive groves and vineyards for the book *The Healing Powers of Olive Oil* reminded me of when I was a kid and our parish priest would drink wine. Not to forget the classic grape fight in *I Love Lucy*'s grape-stomping scene and the many Hallmark Channel romance movies that use wineries as the backdrop to lure you into the picturesque promised land of grape vineyards.

If I was to drink wine, I'd choose Zinfandel from California, which is a medium-dark, dry red wine with blackberry aromas and notes. Ah, and I'd pair it with a scoop of dark chocolate gelato or a chocolate truffle and enjoy the two superfoods. This fantasy may become a reality for my heart and health's sake. So, if you are fascinated by wine, health experts say you can enjoy an occasional glass of wine, but it's advised to stay clear of pesticides and chemicals. Organic wine is recommended. And these days, while I still haven't tasted wine, grapes and grape juice are in my salads and smoothies.

SUPER JUICE, SUPER NUTRIENTS

Buying store-bought all-natural juice without added sugar or juicing it up yourself provides a wealth of nutrients. Take a look at what each different fruit and vegetable juice provides for you. These juices are often offered on restaurant menus and are available at supermarkets and health food stores.

Fresh Juice Type	Nutrients	Why It's Healing
Apple	Fiber, antioxidants	Lowers risk of heart disease
Carrot	Vitamin A	Enhances health of skin, eyes
Cranberry	Vitamin C, phytonutrients, potassium	Boosts immune system, lowers risk of cancer, heart disease
Grape	Antioxidants	Lowers risk of heart disease
Orange	Vitamin C	Enhances immune system, lowers risk of colds, flu, cancer
Pomegranate	Antioxidants	May lower "bad" LDL cholesterol, aids in brain health
Tomato	Lycopene	Lowers risk of developing cancers

Super Energizing Whole-Fruit-and-Vegetable Drink (C-Plus)

This healthful fruit and vegetable juice drink doesn't contain the top 20 superfoods in this book, but it does include a nut milk. Also, the ingredients are easy to find at your supermarket, and not to ignore, you're getting plenty of nutrients. Bottoms up.

1 ounce turnip
1¼ large carrots
3½ ounces pineapple

3 tablespoons almond milk (available at supermarkets)

Juice the carrot and turnip, then pour the juice in a blender, add the pineapple and almond milk and blend well. Pour into a glass and serve immediately.

Makes 1 serving.
(Courtesy: Chiva-Som International Health Resort)

So now you've got one more superfood to meet. Supergrains—good grains. After you check out the super things I'm sharing about whole grains, you may enjoy adding different types to your grocery store basket and combine grains with other superfoods I've introduced.

SUPER-IOR HEALING SUPERFOODS FOR THOUGHT

✓ Other healthy beverages, such as fresh-fruit-infused water, can help keep you hydrated, can energize you, and taste great.

✓ Juice can be good for you if you choose fresh fruit and squeeze it into a juice or if you add an all-natural type of juice into cooking or baking.

✓ Adding fresh fruit juices in smoothies makes these superfood beverages even more nutritious and healthier, and they're an easy way to add more flavor and natural sweetness.

Whole Supergrains (Ancient Oats and Quinoa)

*Oats: A grain, which in England is generally
given to horses, but in Scotland supports the people.*
—SAMUEL JOHNSON, *A Dictionary of the English Language*

Lake Tahoe, where I live, boasts water and nature, which inspire me to continue eating a plant-based, natural diet—including supergrains. During the millennium Y2K panic of 1999, I jumped on the bandwagon and stocked the pantry with whole grains. Brown rice, whole-grain pasta, cereals, crackers, and all-natural granola bars were ready for me and the end of the world as we knew it.

On December 31, New Year's Eve, I crawled into my waterbed with my first senior Brittany spaniel, Dylan, and my orange-and-white cat, Alex. The plan was to watch each country, one by one, go down. Chewing on a granola bar (or two) and sipping bottled water, I watched TV coverage of the New Year gala events, but nothing happened. The world was still intact, and I, a granola girl living in the mountains, had good grains to last for the next century.

These days, when I open a menu at a hotel room faraway, it's super-food items like steel-cut oatmeal with fresh seasonal berries, Belgian waffles with Vermont maple syrup, and Greek yogurt and granola parfait that catch my attention, tease my appetite, and make me feel like I'm at home in California.

THE HISTORY OF WHOLE GRAINS

The history of oats goes back more than four thousand years. Food historians say it may have been available to the Egyptians (but oats were not cultivated) as well as to the Romans and Greeks, who preferred ancient oats instead of wheat. It is believed Marcus Tullius Cicero recommended oats for medicinal use. Also, the Roman author Pliny noted that the Germans grew oats and used it for porridge as a staple in their diet. Ancient quinoa (looks like a grain but is technically a seed) has roots in South America that, like those of oats, go back three thousand to four thousand years, even before Christopher Columbus landed in America.

The Incas and a Quinoa Tale

The supergrain quinoa was the "mother of grains" to the Incas, a tribe of Indians who valued this superfood for its health benefits. As the legend goes, Indians traveled for long journeys while munching on quinoa and fat (in the form of edible "war balls"), most likely for quinoa's energizing benefits. The Incas believed quinoa was the ultimate ancient grain. The seeds of the plant were eaten and considered a primary food source chock-full of nutrients. During planting season, it was said, the Incan leader would plant the first quinoa seed using a gold shovel.

SUPER NUTRIENTS

Oats are chock-full of nutrients, including calcium, iron, magnesium, potassium, protein, and vitamin E. And this is very important, oats contain insoluble fiber and B-glucan, the good stuff that can help lower levels of "bad" cholesterol in the body. Plus, there is no fat or sodium in oats.

Quinoa is touted as a high-protein grain. It also contains lysine (an amino acid). One-half cup of this cooked supergrain boasts eight milligrams of iron—something we all need more of—and five grams of fiber.

HEALTH BENEFITS OF WHOLE GRAINS

A meal combining whole grains (many are infused with fruits, nuts, and seeds) is heart-healthy with a capital *H*. Eating whole grains and fruits is more likely to lower the risk of developing heart disease, and when it comes to protein, plant sources, like nuts and seeds, are linked to a lower risk of heart disease when compared with meat and eggs.[1]

Oats are a superfood without doubt, and medical doctors, nutritionists, and researchers agree. Not only can it help you lower your levels of cholesterol (the fat that can clog arteries), but because it doesn't contain fat or sodium, it may also help reduce your risk of developing heart disease.

And let's not forget that good fiber, which has been linked to lowering the risk of cancer as well as type 2 diabetes. Whole-grain oats are more than just dietary fiber. The B-glucan is touted for its antioxidant and anti-inflammatory benefits. However, more research is needed before any definitive claims are celebrated.[2]

Health-Nut Granola Girl

❖ ❖ ❖

Back in the sixties, a popular hippie health food was granola. It's a cereal mixture of baked oats, nuts, and dried fruit. As time passed, this good-for-you snack made its way to health food stores, and now in the twenty-first century, it's touted in TV commercials and found in bags, boxes, and bins at grocery stores.

When I was a health-conscious nomad between semesters at college, paired with a black Labrador retriever, in Eugene, Oregon, one day a friend gave me a gift to cherish. She allowed me to use her kitchen to make a batch of granola in exchange for walking her Great Dane. Amid a stove, pots, and pans, it took me back to my California days as a kid playing hooky to watch Julia Child on TV with my canine.

I baked a big batch of granola with oats as a base mixed with other superfoods, including dried fruit, nuts, seeds, and maple syrup. The crunchy light-brown clusters were stored inside a plastic container to take with me for survival food, and sweet memories were part of the package.

3 cups old-fashioned rolled oats
½ cup each almonds, pecans, walnuts, roughly chopped
½ cup premium shredded sweet coconut
¼ cup brown sugar
¼ stick of European-style butter, melted
½ cup raw honey
3 tablespoons maple syrup
½ cup each raisins and cranberries

In a pan, place dry ingredients (oats, nuts, coconut, and sugar). Set aside. Mix wet ingredients (butter, honey, syrup) and combine with dry ingredients until all ingredients are coated. Bake in 300 degree F oven 20–25 minutes. Stir a few times. Remove, cool, add dried berries. Store in airtight container in refrigerator.

The kitchen will smell like a cookie shop. A few tips I've learned: less baking time makes a chewier granola, adding dried fruit when the granola is baked is best, easy on the coconut since it's high in fat, and vegetable oil can be used instead of butter. Eating less is more because the contents of these superfoods—nuts and raisins—are rich in fat and calories, but paired with superfood Greek yogurt and/or fruit, this oats-based treat is a superfood.

Makes 8 servings.

Quinoa, like oats, may also help lower the risk of cancer, and it can help beat other ailments, from anemia to fatigue. It can be used for cereals, soups, and rice dishes. While brown rice is a familiar grain, quinoa gets attention in the twenty-first century, and it is a touted superfood throughout the United States and around the world.

While I chose to focus on oats and quinoa, that doesn't mean these are the only two good grains in the world. Adding to the mix are other grains, mostly whole, including barley, bulgur, millet, and rice. (Brown rice has been one of my favorite grains since the seventies.) The more variety of grains you add to your diet, the more variety of vitamins and minerals you'll get, not to forget different textures and flavors, and, well, variety is the spice of good grains!

I'm hardly alone in my love for supergrains. Judy Ridgway, coauthor of *The Olive Oil Diet: Secrets of the Original Superfood*, shares her words of wisdom on oats. "When I was growing up in the north of England, oats were very much part of everyday life. I still enjoy oats today but I use them in a much wider range of dishes than we used to have at home."

She explains that oats can be used in a variety of dishes, including biscuits, breads, breakfast granolas, cakes, crumble toppings, and muffins. "They make an excellent coating for fried fish, vegetable fritters, and fish cakes," adds Ridgway. "Oats are usually sold extra ground or rolled. Ground oatmeal varies in texture from pinhead or steel-cut oatmeal, which is fairly coarse in texture, to quite a fine flour. The latter can sometimes be difficult to find, but it is easy to make at home simply by grinding rolled oats in a food processor until you reach required texture.

"As I have broadened my use of oats I have discovered that they are not only an extremely versatile ingredient but that they are also very healthy. They contain high levels of both soluble and insoluble whole fiber and help to regulate the digestive system," says Ridgway. She adds that the soluble fiber, known as B-glucan, has been shown to reduce the amount of harmful cholesterol in the body and help keep your blood sugar levels steady.

But not all oats are created equal or in one-size-fits-all helpings. If you've got those little convenient packets of instant oatmeal that are chock-full of added sugar, stop right now, especially if you have diabetes. Go for the real old-fashioned oats. It is less processed and higher in fiber so it's the better choice.

Oatmeal is a quick and satisfying breakfast food; however, a fortified whole-grain cereal is nice for a change and gives you essential nutrients, like vitamin D and iron, which if you're busy, aren't getting enough sunshine, or a vegetarian, is something to dish up when you're choosing your whole grains—like this tasty breakfast recipe.

Super Pound-Paring Crunchy French Toast and Seasonal Berries

A story often told to me by a couple devoted to one another is linked to ancient grains, sort of. I used to clean their home when I was in graduate school, and one morning in between my rounds in the six bedrooms, I was invited to a hot breakfast. The man said to me, "I married Edith because she is an excellent cook." He laughed and she blushed.

Instead of a bowl of oatmeal (a staple breakfast for another elderly and active couple I worked for), I was served a plate of French toast and a generic brand of store-bought syrup. (The bread was white and cooked the old-school way without the crunch.) As I ate, the man forewarned me of the perils of being single. This old-time popular dish, with my own reworked recipe inspired by the long-time married duo, is one to love. I did change it up with whole grains and fresh berries (blueberries to preserve my eyes during spinsterhood in my golden years).

2 organic brown eggs	Maple syrup, premium
½ cup 2-percent milk or	(Crown Maple,
half-and-half	cinnamon infused)
1 teaspoon cinnamon	Confectioners' sugar
1 teaspoon vanilla	(optional)
1 cup whole-grain cereal	Fresh fruit (blueberries
(General Mills Total)	and raspberries)
2–3 slices whole-grain	Almonds, sliced
bread	Mint sprigs for garnish
1 tablespoon European-	
style butter (extra for	
topping toast)	

In a bowl, whisk eggs, milk, cinnamon, and vanilla. Set aside. On a flat dish or pan, crush cereal. Dip bread into egg mixture, then in cereal until both sides of bread are coated. In a frying pan, melt butter. Place bread into hot pan. Cook a few minutes and turn. Once light brown and crispy, remove. Put toasted bread onto a serving dish. Add a pat of butter, drizzle syrup on top. Dust with sugar. Add berries. Cut in half or triangles. Garnish with almonds and mint. The whole-grain flakes and nuts are crunchy and full of texture and flavor you'll cherish like nature's gift or your mother and father.

Makes 2–3 servings.

Congratulations! You've completed my crash course on 20 super-foods (with some sidekicks). Now, whip up a smoothie and come with me into the Fountain of Youth. I'll take you to another place to show

how these same favorite foods, my chosen ones, are going to be your best friends throughout your life (whether you're twenty-five, fifty, or seventy-five) by allowing you to fool the aging process and stall Father Time.

SUPER-IOR HEALING SUPERFOODS FOR THOUGHT

✓ Ancient grains—all types—may help lower the risk of bad cholesterol, boost immunity, and much more.

✓ Supergrains, including oats, quinoa, brown rice, and whole-grains in bread, are touted as "heart healthy" by food product manufacturers.

✓ Consuming whole grains every day is a super way to fill up and not out, which can help you maintain a healthy weight for you.

✓ And if you get and stay lean, it can lower your risk of obesity-linked diseases, such as heart disease, cancer, and diabetes.

PART 3

THE SUPERFOODS OF YOUTH

CHAPTER

2 3

Age-Defying Superstuff

Grow old along with me!
The best is yet to be.
—ROBERT BROWNING, "Rabbi ben Ezra"

The Y2K incident was a good preparedness adventure thanks to my squirrel-stocking emergency mode to get water and supergrains in the pantry. (The exercise was antiaging.) Being a baby boomer who defied anyone over thirty while growing up with challenges, it's part of my age-defying roots to shun junk food and stay active—two antics to help me age gracefully—at home or on the road.

In my forties, seeking a soul mate in the mountain environment, I ended up meeting a man I connected with online. We met at the local casino at Lake Tahoe. I brought my younger sibling for moral support. He went ahead to scrutinize the younger man for me—"the perfectionist diva." The report: "He looks scruffy, like Ralph, that old cat you rescued." I decided to play the odds and joined Ralphie II for dinner, as planned. I ordered a shrimp louie and sipped tea; my date, ten years my junior, smoked cigarettes and swallowed manly drinks—whiskey. It wasn't a *Terms of Endearment* classic film post-meal-and-drinks love connection on the beach or a *Green Card* movie of opposites attracting and falling in like. While being mateless sometimes is lonely, not having a like-minded health-conscious partner was a deal breaker for me that night. One doggie bag later, I shared fish remnants at home with my devoted feline, who still had nine lives to go.

Defying Aging with Superfoods

Whether we're solo or not, from the day we are born, it's inevitable we all age. So, whatever generation you are in—millennial, generation X, baby boomer, traditionalist—superfoods and their healing powers may help you age gracefully and live a longer, healthier life. From head to toe, I've provided some health issues that may affect people as they grow older. While superfoods are not a cure-all or miracle, if incorporated in the diet early on they very well may be key to living a healthier, longer, quality life with less aches and pains. Read on.

ARTHRITIS

When the joints start to degenerate, stiffness and pain and lack of mobility come into play. Think of *The Wizard of Oz*'s Tin Man. When his legs and arms were not oiled, it was difficult for him to walk with ease.

Super Antiaging Tips: You may not have stiff joints. This may be due to genes, exercise, and luck. As we age, low-impact exercise such as swimming and walking the dog, and drinking water and tea may be helpful. Research shows that gentle exercising, such as yoga or swimming using breaststrokes and sidestrokes, may provide relief for arthritis.

Favorite Superfoods Rx: Vitamin C, the antioxidant vitamin, is necessary to build bone (lemons, berries), vitamin D may help lessen inflammation and calcification of the joints, and omega-3 acids are important for lubrication of joints; it also reduces proinflammatory chemicals called prostaglandins (shellfish).

BRAIN HEALTH

Alzheimer's disease, Parkinson's disease, depression, and dementia. Symptoms can vary, but memory loss, confusion, and deterioration of the mind can result.

Super Antiaging Tips: While you may have inherited your aunt's amazing gift of memory, it could also be due to your lifestyle. I always say it's essential to tend to my "writer's brain" (working it so I don't lose it) and to try and guard my brain wellness; diet is not excluded.

Favorite Superfoods Rx: Some doctors believe that a diet high in essential fatty acids is brain food. Because the brain is composed of fat, the more good fats in the diet, the better for the cell membrane function in the brain (shellfish). Also, antioxidant-rich vegetables may help get rid of damaging free radical scavengers, which may be helpful for brain wellness (blueberries, greens, cruciferous vegetables, potatoes, and sea vegetables).

According to research, blueberries seemed to slow and even reverse many of the degenerative diseases associated with aging. Scientists at the U.S. Department of Agriculture's Human Nutrition Research Center on Aging found that blueberries—rich in vitamins A and C and other nutrients—have functional antioxidants and anti-inflammatory effects on the brain and muscle tissue.

Interestingly, maple syrup comes to mind when preserving our memory and staving off Alzheimer's disease. An extract of the sticky sweet stuff stopped the dangerous folding in different types of brain proteins, according to research findings from the Krembil Institute of the University of Toronto in Canada. Lab studies show it's the antioxidant-fighting activity of the phenolic extracts of maple syrup that produce neuroprotective effects similar to those of the resveratrol found in red wine and grape juice.

EYES

Dry eyes and nearsightedness or farsightedness can occur at any age. But cataracts, glaucoma, and macular degeneration are more apt to happen as we age; however, superfoods can come to the rescue.

Super Anti-Aging Tips: I had put off an eye exam for years. One night, after a long day on the computer, I glanced at the TV and the words were blurry on the screen. That was spooky! One eye exam later: no eye diseases, no prescription eye glasses prescribed. The optometrist gave credit to good genes. I was advised to turn down the brightness setting and to take eye breaks while working on the computer, and there's more to nourish the eyes.

Favorite Superfoods Rx: The consensus is, vitamins A, C, and E and the mineral selenium are important for good eye health. People who maintain inadequate levels of these antioxidants and selenium are at high risk. The top 20 superfoods are helpful because many of them contain some of these nutrients.

Vitamin A: broccoli, crab, eggs, kale, spinach, sweet potatoes; **Vitamin C:** broccoli, cauliflower, kale, lemon, strawberries; **Vitamin E:** almonds, kale, hazelnuts, peanuts; **Selenium:** Brazil nuts, chicken breast, cottage cheese, lobster, scallops, shrimp.

BONES

Osteoporosis, or the brittle bone disease, can happen at any age and to both women and men. But as we grow older our bones are more prone to bone density loss.

Super Antiaging Tips: If you are a Caucasian woman and petite, like me, we both may be at higher risk for bone loss, according to the facts. But on the upside, I've never broken a bone—not one. I did dislocate a kneecap, but it healed quickly and gave me an adventure story to tuck away. It happened while camping, during roughhousing. I'll never forget seeing my kneecap pop out of my leg, nor the ride in an ambulance, but I survived. The lesson: Don't take bones—or any part connected to them—for granted.

Favorite Superfoods Rx: Consuming an adequate intake of calcium and vitamin D is good for bones (broccoli, cheese, Greek yogurt, ice cream). Eating a vitamin-and-mineral fortified whole-grain cereal and drinking calcium- and vitamin D–enriched milk are helpful to ensure bone-boosting protection, too.

A Gallery of Superfoods Photos

Some of these photos show recipes that are included in this book. Other images combine favorite superfoods to inspire you to create your own superfoods recipes.

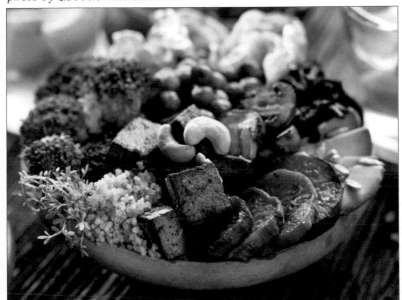

Versatile, flavorful superfoods appeal to a wide range of tastes and diets, from vegans to fish and fowl lovers. Shown here: Buddha bowl of mixed vegetables, grains, and nuts; seafood soup with mussels and crab.

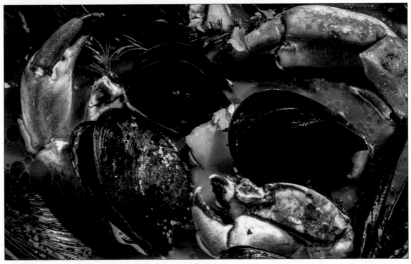

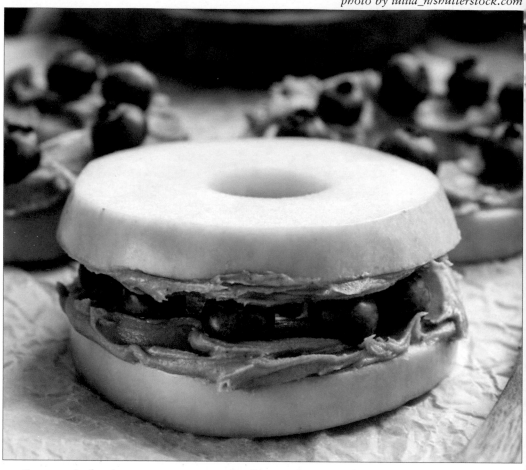

For a superfood treat, try green apple slices with peanut butter and blueberries . . . or get creative with toppings on avocado toast.

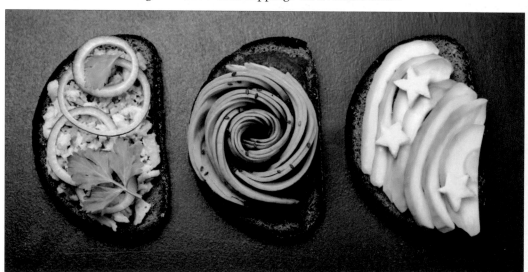

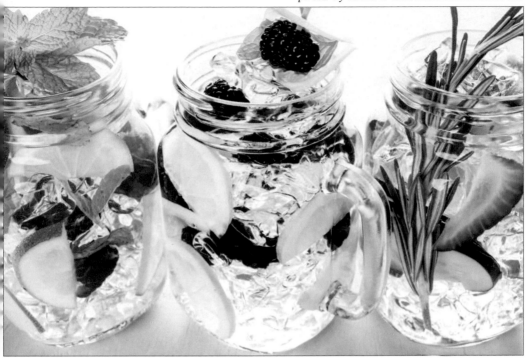

Enjoy refreshing infused water and fruit juices to stay healthfully hydrated.

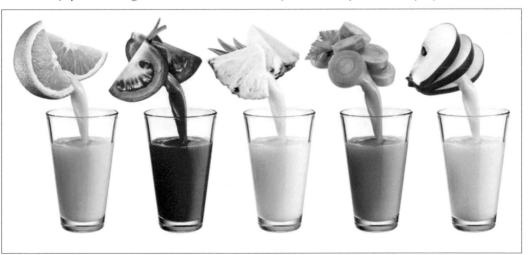

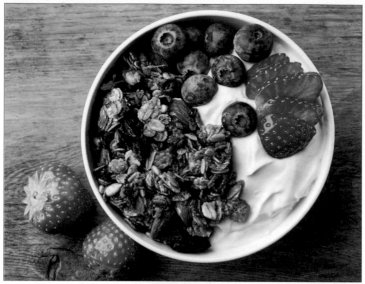

Start your day with a superfood breakfast, such as a yogurt parfait, an apple oatmeal muffin, or whole-wheat pancakes topped with natural maple syrup.

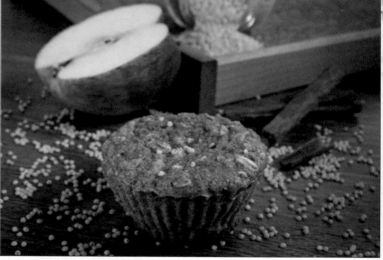

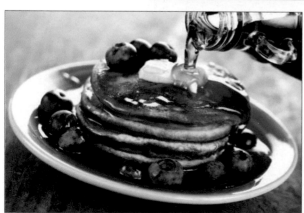

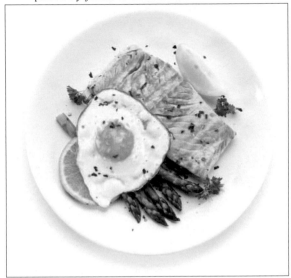

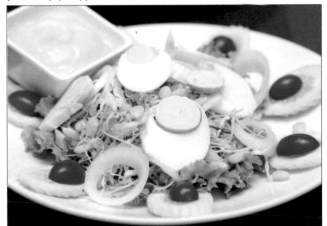

Eggs are an excellent source
of protein whether eaten by
themselves or paired with other
superfoods. Hard-boiled eggs
add protein to salads and are
not fattening!

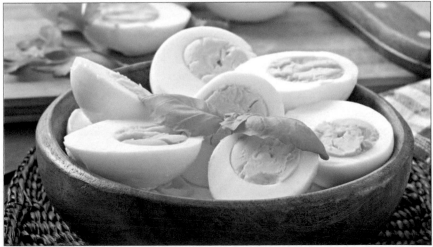

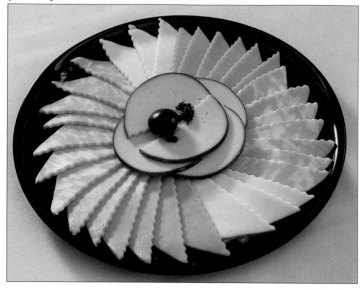

Cheeses and nuts contain essential nutrients for our mental and physical well-being. Nut butters now go far beyond peanut butter to include pistachio, cashew, and hazelnut butters.

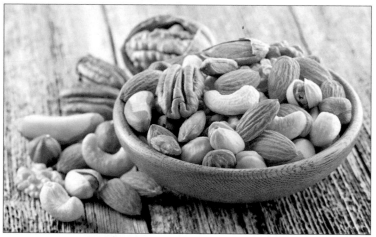

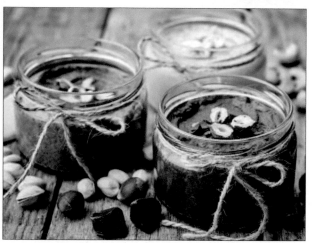

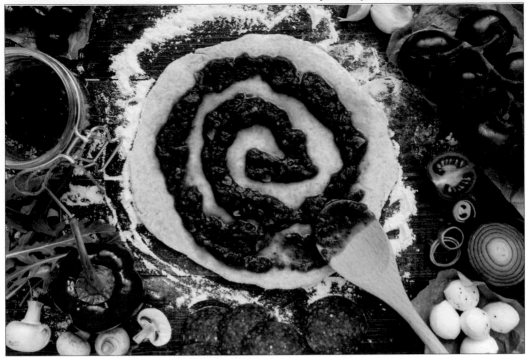

Make your own superfood pizza using whole-wheat dough,
fresh tomatoes, feta cheese, and basil.

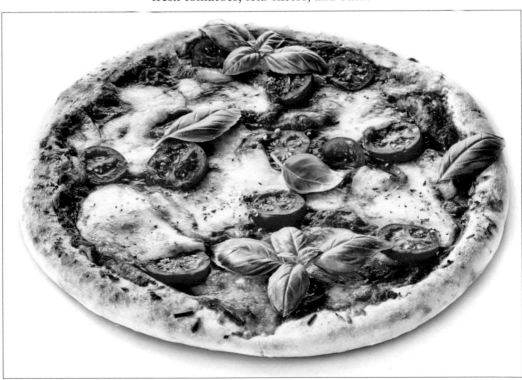

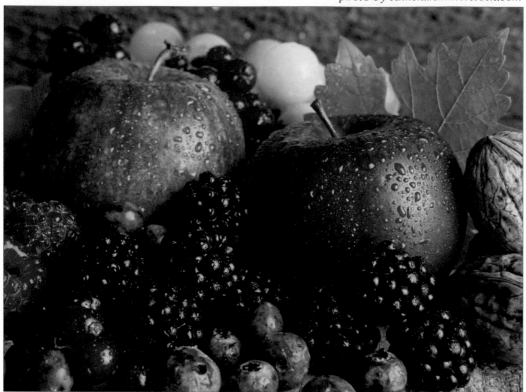

Apples, blackberries, melons . . . all fruits are delicious superfoods
that can be enjoyed raw or cooked, alone or in combination.

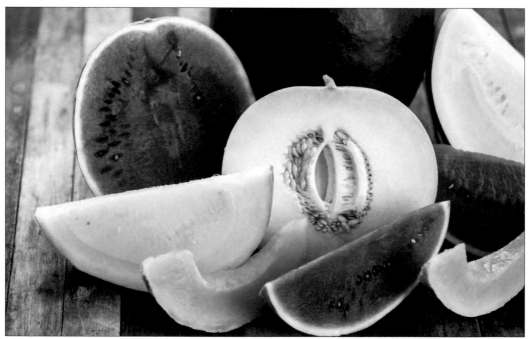

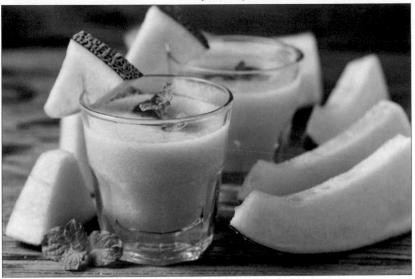

Smoothies can be made from your favorite fruits and vegetables. Add nutty butters or all-natural gelato or ice cream to make smoothies super creamy and protein-rich.

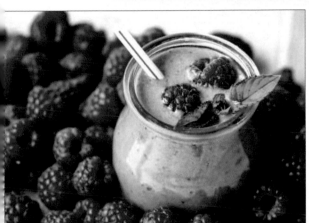

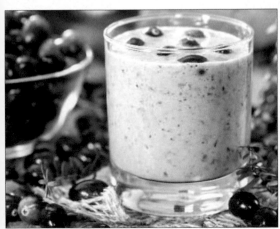

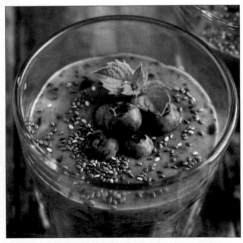

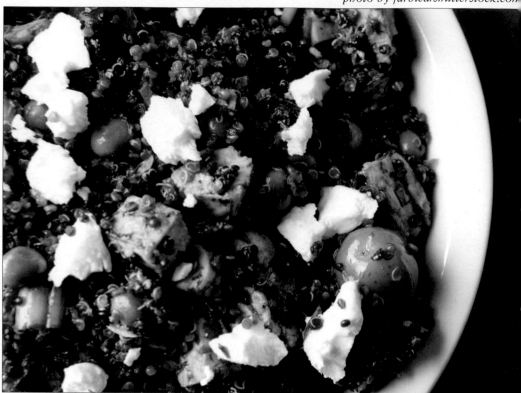

Colorful salads combining ancient grains with greens or root vegetables are heart-healthy and full of vitamins. Shown here: red beet, quinoa, and chicken salad; avocado, tomato, chickpeas, spinach, and cucumber salad.

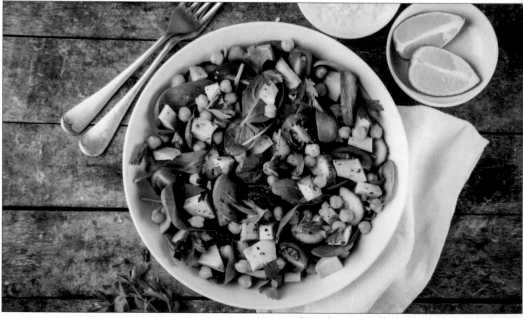

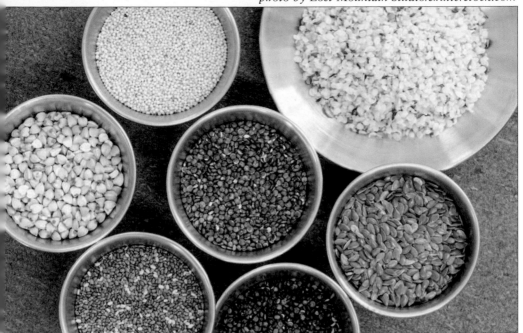

Ancient grains and healthy organic edible seeds offer a bounty of health benefits. Enjoy cooked mixed ancient grains cereal for a satisfying meal any time of day . . . or combine grains with other superfoods to create a farm-fresh healthy organic summer salad like this one with quinoa, chickpeas, feta, cucumber, and tomato.

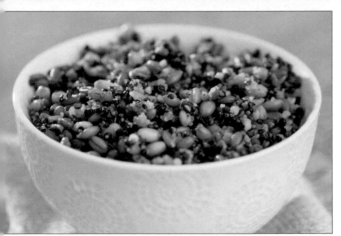

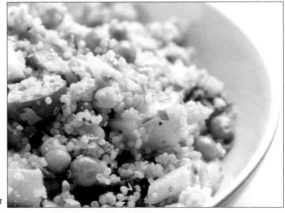

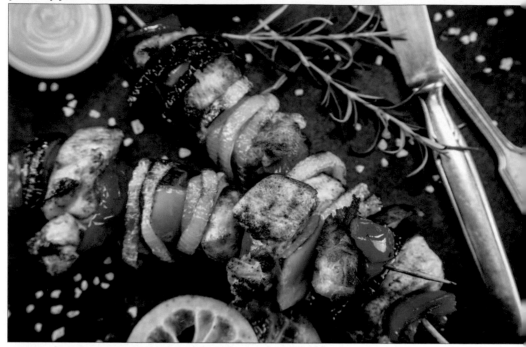

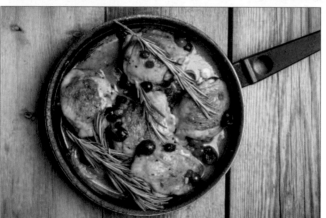

Grill it, bake it, broil it . . . poultry is one of the most versatile of the superfoods. Shown here: chicken kebabs with vegetables; pan-roasted chicken with cranberries and rosemary; traditional roast turkey with superfood garnish.

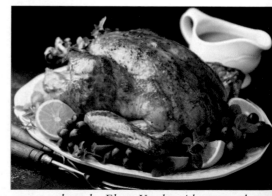

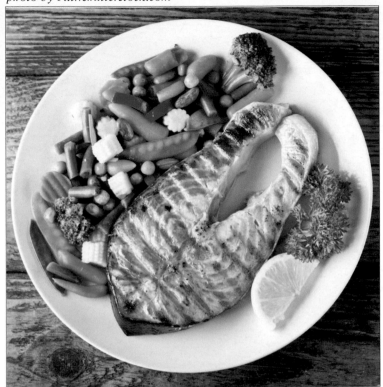

Fatty fish contains heart-healthy omega-3 fatty acids and provides protein, calcium, selenium, and other minerals. Shown here: salmon with vegetable medley; halibut with vegetable medley.

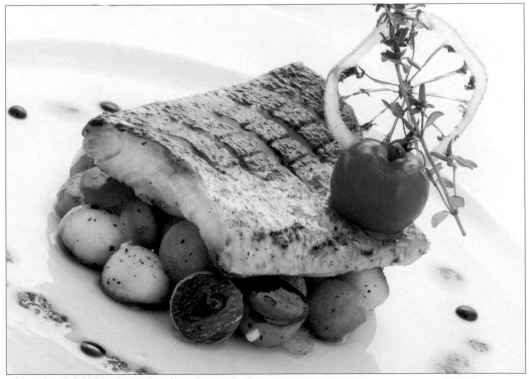

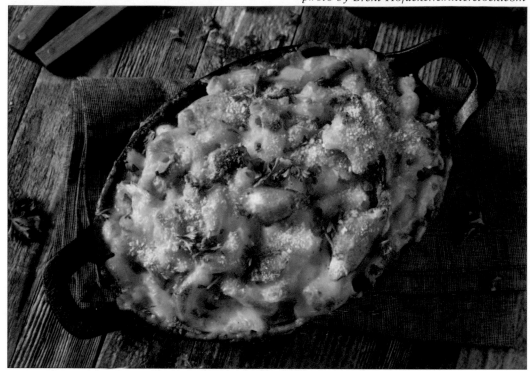

Nature's bounty from the sea can be prepared in countless ways.
Have you ever tried mac 'n' cheese with lobster?

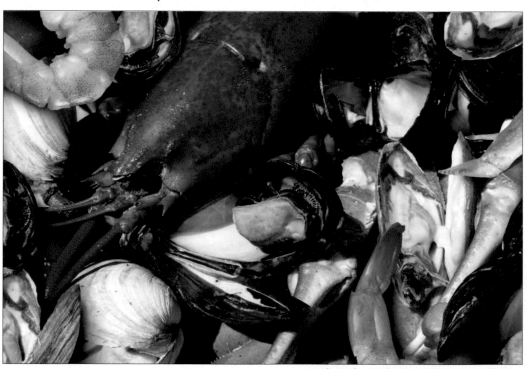

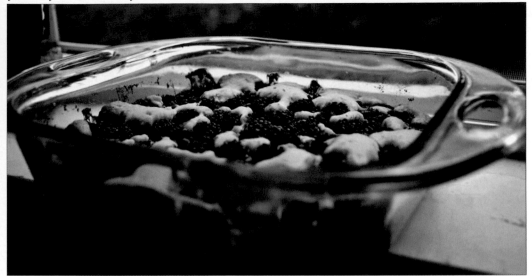

No need to skip dessert
when you can choose
superfood treats such
as boysenberry cobbler
topped with a dollop
of all-natural ice cream
or a slice of apple crumble.
And how about a scoop
of pumpkin gelato?

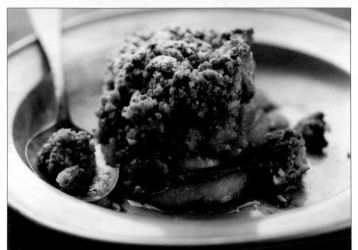

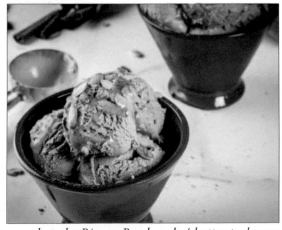

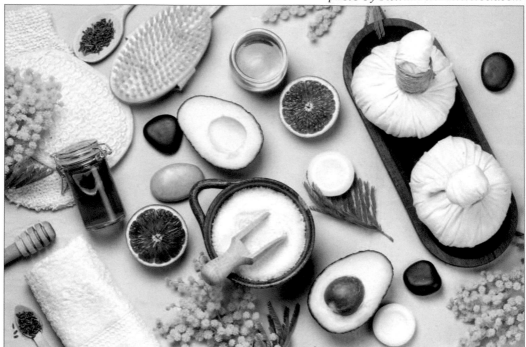

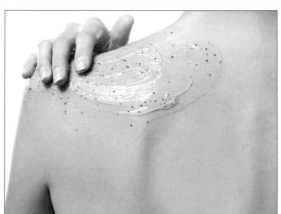

Beauty products made from superfoods are featured in top spas—and you can make them at home.

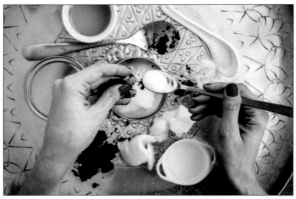

Calcium-rich yogurt can help you maintain strong bones. If your body is deficient in calcium, the body will steal it from your bones. This weakens your skeleton and can lead to brittle bone disease, which does affect older people but can happen no matter what your age is and in both men and women.

TEETH

Your pearly whites are essential to good overall health and well-being. In the twenty-first century, dentistry is progressive and maintaining your smile is easier as we age than ever before.

Super Anti-Aging Tips: Not everyone aspired to be a dental hygienist, like I did, but it may have helped me to try to stay on top of dental care throughout the years as our bodies (and hormones) change, affecting dental care. Tending to my teeth and gums (and those of my companion animals) is one of the things on my must-do list for health's sake and peace of mind. Regular brushing, flossing, and dental visits and cleanings are part of the good dental hygiene package, but there is more you can do at home, too.

Favorite Superfoods Rx: Calcium is an important mineral that protects your teeth (cheese, Greek yogurt). Vitamin C is an antioxidant that keeps your gums healthy (broccoli, berries, lemons, and water).

SUPERFOODS FOR EVERY GENERATION

At every age we need superfoods. But it seems that for each generation the choices of superfoods differ. A lot. Age matters and can influence superfood choices. But superfood favorites (or not) also can depend on where people live, too.

The Midwest may not have access to fresh fruit and vegetables year-round, like the West Coast does. Fast-food choices may be more popular than superfoods in the Deep South. But in their defense, the Gulf States have their pick of fresh shellfish, much like the Pacific Northwest and the New England states.

Wherever you live and whatever your age, favorite superfoods— whole, natural foods—are growing more in demand around the nation and globe. And yes, there are ways to get your fill of superfoods to fill the void of what you may be lacking. If fresh fruit and vegetables are not available, frozen and canned are available. Nuts and seeds are fine as dried superfoods. Greek yogurt, cheese, and gelato are good to go in their frozen state. And Northeastern/Canadian maple syrup to live for has a long shelf life and can be enjoyed wherever you are.

Here, take a look at the choices people in each age group make, why they make them, and what they do to stay on top of their superfoods throughout the years.

Gen Z, iGen, or Centennials (Born 1996 and later): The new generation of young people (from toddlers to teens) has been introduced to superfoods (functional foods that are organic, all natural, no preservatives, additives, chemicals) by more mainstream food companies, big and small, because of the turning of the tide for going back to nature for health's sake. In the twenty-first century, it is "in" to eat clean, fresh, and real food. Favorite superfoods: blueberries, eggs, oats, and yogurt.

Millennials or Gen Y (Born 1977–1995): Welcome to the adventurous millennials. When it comes to eating, this generation is bold, and they go for exciting superfoods. Diverse flavors and textures and fresh to spicy tastes are some of the things this generation likes. Not only do they take risks and like to eat global cuisine from different cultures, they also cook it up, too. Favorite superfoods: exotic smoothies, kale, sea vegetables, and seeds.

Generation X, Gen Xers (Born 1965–1976): The boomers' children are in a good place. As the offspring of baby boomers, they were introduced to natural foods—not the convenience fare the boomers were fed. Instead of eating processed food from a box or a can, they are more apt to buy whole, fresh food and shop at supercenters to get it or perhaps even grow their own produce. Favorite superfoods: all-natural smoothies, juice drinks, sushi, and protein shakes and bars.

Baby Boomers (Born 1946–1964): Age-conscious, health-minded boomers do whatever they can to stay younger and enjoy a longer lifespan than their parents did. That means going vegetarian or vegan, eating heart-healthy foods, antioxidant-rich and fiber-plentiful fruits and vegetables, and good fats found in superfoods. This active generation can be found foraging at farmer's markets and growing gardens. Plus, the young-at-heart boomers are fans of farm-to-table restaurants and home cooking to get clean food minus the processed junk and chemicals. Favorite superfoods: fruits, Greek yogurt, whole grains, and vegetables.

Traditionalists (Born 1945 and before): The elderly people in the twenty-first century are living longer lives of greater quality than ever before. While superfoods are available, sometimes convenience foods and fast foods (often processed) may be a lure because they're easy to prepare and foods in a box or a can last longer. But premade food (popular in the twentieth century after World War II) often is laden with salt, sugar, flavorings, and preservatives and is not as healthful as clean superfoods. Favorite superfoods: Chicken, potatoes, ice cream, pasta.

Future Generations (Born 2019 and onward): When I wrote the book *Doctors' Orders*, supplements were the primary focus, but many doctors talked superfoods and I listened. Dr. Robert Roundtree discussed kid-friendly superfoods that can help enhance longevity, such as berries (blueberries, raspberries, strawberries), which are rich in antioxidants and support the immune system by neutralizing free radicals; green leafy vegetables (spinach, kale), which are a good source of folic acid (B vitamin) and good for the maturation of bone marrow and as a preventative for cancer and heart disease; cruciferous vegetables (broccoli, cabbage), which provide glucosinolates, which are sulfur-containing compounds that help the liver detoxify chemicals.[1]

No matter what age you are, including superfoods in your daily diet can help you lower the risk of developing chronic ailments and age-related diseases, which may be due to genes and environment.

Super Youth-Boosting Veggie-Fruit Smoothie Immune Aid

Here is a healthy savory smoothie that includes age-defying nutrients. To stall the aging process, it's important to keep our immune system stoked to stave off colds (which can escalate into bronchitis or pneumonia) and inflammation (a culprit of age-related diseases). It's chock-full of fresh superfoods and a super spice and herb—antiaging garlic, a super boost that may require an acquired taste.

1½ large carrots
½ ounce beetroot (juice
   and powder available
   online)

⅔-inch piece ginger
1 red apple
1 garlic clove

Juice all of the ingredients, including carrots, beetroot, ginger, apple, and garlic. Pour into a glass and serve immediately.

Makes 1 serving.
(Courtesy: Chiva-Som International Health Resort)

Aging gracefully can help you feel and look your best, as can staying fit and lean for your personal best. Moving on (pun intended), my favorite superfoods can help you to get and/or stay at your best weight and size. Find out how exactly these superfoods can help you to stay clear of gaining unwanted body fat and pounds.

SUPER-IOR HEALING SUPERFOODS FOR THOUGHT

✓ You can take years off your body and mind by changing your diet—and that means adding functional foods to your lifestyle.

✓ The superfoods picks in this book may help you gain muscle mass and lose body fat as well as stay on top of the aging game (no matter if you're twenty-five or seventy-five).

✓ Antioxidant-rich superfoods may also help you lower your risk of developing age-related cancers as the odds increase as your birthdays come and go.

✓ Heart-healthy superfoods—like the top 20 favorites—can help you maintain healthy blood pressure numbers, cholesterol levels, and blood sugar numbers, which may stave off type 2 diabetes, heart disease, and even cancer.

Skinny Superfoods

*The healthy man is the thin man. But you don't
need to go hungry for it; remove the flours, starches
and sugars; that's all.*
    —SAMAEL AUN WEOR

Before an early autumn trip to the Pacific Northwest, I wanted to dump five pounds. For a week, I ate a semi–Stone Age diet: leafy greens, nuts, seeds, and fruit; no catching fish or fowl at the lake for me. It worked. At Sea-Tac Airport late one evening, I was standing in size 4 skinny jeans, two tee shirts, two sweaters, a thick coat, neck scarf, and combat boots. I was lean, layered, and cool, right? Wrong.

Shocked by the crowd of people, I felt like a creature from another planet. Seattle locals and visitors were dressed in Hawaiian shirts, shorts, and thongs. I looked like I was transported to the wrong terminal. One man asked me, "Are you going to Alaska?" Embarrassed, I answered, "Nah, Vancouver. I don't like to lug a heavy carry-on bag." And in my mind, I justified my reasoning that because I'm small, it's easier to bundle up in clothes (leggings, jeans, tees, and sweaters), carry less. And that's why I played the get-skinny-and-layer game with credit to the superfoods cavewoman diet. Note to self: Savor skinny superfoods for their amazing pounds-off powers but forego piling on clothes when going to a destination known for its warm Mediterranean climate.

Each time you savor skinny superfoods, like I did before that trip, and you have a goal to drop unwanted pounds, turn to filling, nutrient-rich, low-cal foods. These superfoods are a natural remedy to help you take it off effortlessly. Superfoods in the morning, afternoon, and night can give you energy, help fight fat, and are truly a dieter's best friend. Nutritionists at health spas will tell you that they serve water-dense fresh fruits and vegetables because they can help dieters fill up but not out—much like drinking tea.

SKINNY SUPERFOODS

Top medical experts, including Dr. Mehmet Oz (seen interviewing nutrition-minded guests about superfoods, from seeds to watermelons, in a variety of TV show segments) confirm certain superfoods may boost body fat loss. Plus, the celeb doctor even had his own book on superfoods, *Food Can Fix It*, published in 2017.

The healthy, "fat-burning" or "fat-melting" or "metabolism-boosting" superfoods include nutrient-dense fruits and vegetables, according to my years of writing articles on this topic, past and present. I have been called the "skinny writer" by magazine and newspaper editors who published my writings.

Back in the late twentieth century, we didn't call the skinny foods superfoods (well maybe once I did do that), but *fat-melting foods, fat-blasting foods*, or *fat-burning foods* were the key phrases for the best foods to lose unwanted body fat and pounds. And now, in the present day, we have studies using the word *superfoods* that show exactly how these foods can help you to dump the weight.

SUPER FAT BURNERS

Past research proves compounds in superfoods can boost your metabolism (calorie-burning power). Also, medical researchers believe that compounds in superfoods such as apples, berries, citrus, and melons can help blast belly fat. The ongoing research shows that certain antioxidants, such as catechins, may be some of the fat-fighters. And there's more . . .

There are also other ways superfoods can help you lose unwanted weight. Low-calorie, low-fat, water-dense foods can fill you up—not out. You'll fight fat effortlessly, graze on minimeals, and not be hungry or crave processed foods. The more you eat natural, nutrient-dense, clean superfoods, consuming cakes, cookies, burgers, and chips will seem less desirable and more like history for you.

And don't forget that plenty of fruits and vegetables—not unhealthy, empty-of-nutrition food choices—are healing superfoods with remarkable powers for your body, mind, and spirit.

Years ago, medical doctors I interviewed taught me everything I needed to know about super fat burners. I was told they were nothing fancy or pricey—just nature's wonder foods that can help you get rid of unwanted fat. Many of the superfoods, or "super fat burners," are low in calories (especially fruits, vegetables, and even whole grains), so you can eat them in unlimited portions and lose pounds.

Not only do superfoods negate their own calories, but they also burn off calories from other foods. For instance, when you top whole-grain pasta with tomatoes, the pasta's complex carbs will increase your calorie-burning power.

A PLANT-BASED DIET WORKS WONDERS

Diet doctors whom I've talked to throughout three decades agree that a meatless (or almost) diet is the ultimate for fat burning. We know, as noted above, that grain, fruits, and vegetables are modest in calories and fill you up, not out. (I learned that a plant-based diet was the best weight loss diet as a teenager. As I began to rebel and stop eating the meat entrees my mom served on the weekends and wolfing down burgers at fast-food chains, losing weight wasn't an issue, nor was I hungry.)

So, you may argue "I need protein!" I agree. But switching eggs, fish, legumes, nuts, and poultry (in moderation) for meat can make a big difference in maintaining your ideal weight. Losing weight by eating complex-carb-rich foods can and does work.

I'm hardly alone. Millions of people who eat a plant-based diet don't count calories or worry about portions. We build our meals around negative-calorie fruits and vegetables. Think salads, veggies, stir-fries, and soups and sandwiches. You'll increase your body's calorie- and fat-burning potential while you enjoy carb-rich foods that trigger hormones that signal your metabolism to speed up and burn more fat.

TOP 10 SKINNY SUPERFOODS

So, eating skinny superfoods can help you to get and stay leaner at any age, but some foods may help you to lose unwanted body fat and pounds a bit faster and easier. They include fat-burning foods such as fruits and vegetables. Some of these foods fill you up and work while you're at a resting state. I can personally attest that at least half of these foods—from the top 20 superfoods list—help get rid of water retention, some more than others.

Here, take a look at a few of my past and present favorite tried and true superfoods that may be your best friends. (I'm excluding nuts, seeds, fish, and poultry because in moderation these foods are diet friendly, but not as much as these following chosen picks.) These super fat-fighting superfoods are my personal favorites to lose pounds, fast and easy.

APPLES

Apples are full of deliciousness. This fruit is a rich source of fiber that plumps up food as it's digested, report researchers in past research. The plumping up increases satiety so you feel satisfied.

Also, emotional and stress eating habits often can lead to eating unhealthy comfort foods, whereas a crunchy apple is a wholesome, natural stress-fighting superfood. It is low in calories, fat, and cholesterol. What's more, thanks to the fiber in apples, these superfruits can help you stay regular and more energized, and that can help in weight loss, too.

Did you know munching on an apple every day may not only keep the doctor away but stave off unwanted weight, too? Scientists at Washington State University have found compounds in Granny Smith apples that may help disorders related to obesity. The findings, published in the journal *Food Chemistry*, show those crunchy, tart green apples rank highest in nondigestible compounds that create a balance of bacteria in the colon and metabolic processes that help fill you up, not out.[1]

BERRIES

Another fat-burning superfruit is the berry—all types. Throughout my years writing about diet and nutrition, nutritionists and medical doctors have touted the benefits of fiber-rich berries, which (like apples) help to reduce absorption of fat and calories.

As explained in chapter 4, which covers berries and avocados, all of these sweet and tart babies are nutrient dense, which is a godsend when you're shedding unwanted weight. Berries are diet friendly since they are low in fat and calories and are cholesterol free and sweet, so if you have a sweet tooth, berries can nip your urge to grab a donut or candy bar by replacing it with a bowl of berries or a berry smoothie.

Blueberries, for instance, help your body burn fat. These little dark-blue superfruits are chock-full of dietary fiber, which helps reduce your absorption of fat and calories. Plus, blueberries are rich in vitamin A and C, both super to your health when cutting calories. One cup of these berries contains fewer than 100 calories.

CRUCIFERS

Broccoli, cauliflower, and kale—three super vegetables in the high-fiber cabbage family that are known as fat fighters, like apples and berries. This mighty trio is one that may take a while to like its taste, but once you do, because they're low in fat and fill you up, you may learn to love the flavor.

By mixing and matching broccoli, cauliflower, and kale with bell peppers, carrots, mushrooms, and dark-green lettuce, such as spinach and romaine (not to leave out herbs and spices), you'll increase their texture and flavor, and eat more fat-fighting super vegetables. A baby broccoli side dish complete with red onion and red bell pepper, and drizzled with olive oil and a bit of real butter will not taste like bunny food!

GREEK YOGURT

Nope, yogurt is not a superfruit or vegetable, but it does have super benefits that can help you stay on the dieting track. Since it is high in calories and high in fat, less is more. Mixing it up with apples or berries can give you plenty of filling fiber but also calcium, which studies show can calm you and help curb cravings and fight stress eating, which will make losing unwanted weight easier.

Fat-free yogurt may be lower in calories and lower in fat, but it's not real food, and for me, it's just not satisfying. However, super creamy plain yogurt drizzled with raw honey is a comfort food like ice cream, and it's a super source of calcium.

LEMONS

Instead of touting popular oranges, lemons are another superfruit that are often on a dieter's menu and for good reason. Like apples, lemons (also grapefruit and oranges) are a super source of filling fiber. But versatile lemons also can help burn fat as well as be detoxifying, and research studies as well as medical doctors' experience prove it.

Back when I was a nutrition-diet columnist for a variety of health magazines, I recall the popular lemony "master cleanse" shared with me by Northern California–based Elson M. Haas, M.D. He explained to me the wonders of nature's simple detoxifying beverage concoction, which included 2 tablespoons of fresh lemon juice, 1 tablespoon of maple syrup, $\frac{1}{10}$ tablespoon of cayenne pepper, and eight ounces of water. Drink eight to ten glasses a day.

He told me he would join some of his patients to help cleanse the body and dump unwanted weight. Since I love lemons—sweet and tart—and I love water, I was curious; still I didn't try the juice cleanse diet.

POTATOES

Both russet and sweet potatoes can help you lose unwanted weight like superfruits. One reason is that they are full of potassium, which can counteract sodium and reduce water retention, nutritionists will tell you. Potatoes are low in calories, fat, and sodium. The fiber content can be filling, and the carbohydrate fix is calming if you're looking for a stress-eating food.

Studies have shown that eating starchy complex carbohydrates—like a potato—revs up the mood-boosting brain chemical serotonin, which works to lessen hunger pangs. Top a hot baked tater with cruciferous vegetables and Parmesan cheese for more vitamins, minerals, and flavor. Not only will it help you take off unwanted pounds, you'll also enjoy the comfort food without a lot of trouble putting it together.

SPINACH

Raw spinach, another super vegetable, is an ideal slimming superfood. It's low in fat and calories, it's filling, and with lettuce can help wash away fat. Spinach salad mixes are nutrient dense, and served in satisfying, meal-sized portions, can be the path to quicker weight loss.

Also, spinach contains magnesium—a mineral that can help you sleep better. Research shows when people are sleep deprived, mindless eating can happen as they try to get energy and a wakeful state, whereas a good night's rest may be all your body craves—not food. Since both spinach and lettuce are high volume foods, they are a dieter's godsend—low in calories, no fat, and when drizzled with vinegar and a bit of olive oil they are full of disease-fighting antioxidants.

Mixing it up (as I discuss in chapter 6, the chapter on leafy greens) is not only tastier, but you get other perks, too. Kale is also rich in fiber, like raw spinach, and water, too, so like all of these slimming foods it fills you up. By eating high-fiber vegetables like spinach, you'll consume fewer calories throughout the day because your stomach will be full, thanks to the fat-burning superfood.

TOMATOES

Eating a salad of dark leafy greens paired with juicy, fresh tomatoes, another versatile superfood, can help you drop unwanted pounds, too. Tomatoes—all kinds, Roma, cherry, heirloom, and more—lower the production of the hormone insulin, which locks fat in the fat cells. This, in turn, results in less fat being stored in your body. Also, tomatoes contain pectin, a type of dietary fiber that has been shown by past research to help you feel full.

Fresh tomatoes (my mother used canned a lot) contain mostly carbohydrates and water. So, like all these skinny superfoods, they are low-calorie, low-fat, and carb-rich foods that are satisfying and can curb hunger pangs as well as cravings for processed, unhealthy foods.

When I'm at the Salt Lake City airport, I always order spicy tomato salsa—a known fat-burning superfood—and warm chips with a nice crunch at a restaurant. Tomato salsa with jalapeno peppers or chilies may boost your calorie-burning power. Plus, it is low in calories and fat. It's not heavy for a flight, and it fills me up, not out. It's a tradition for me to order tomato salsa with a cup of hot chamomile tea.

WATER

Instead of indulging in food when you're stressed out (you may not even be hungry), try reaching for a glass of water (including herbal tea); sip it and have it with you wherever you are. Not only does water keep your body running properly from head to toe and keep your vital organs healthy while you're dealing with life's ups and downs, but it also doesn't have calories or fat, and it can help curb cravings and fill you up when you do eat so you'll eat less rather than more.

Because many of us, including myself from time to time, confuse hunger with thirst, it's a super idea to drink bottled water or a cup of tea before you reach for a snack. You may be surprised that you're not hungry at all and almost were fooled by mindless eating. It's also a super idea to drink a glass of fat-burning water or iced tea before a meal to help fill up and not be tempted to overeat (that's what doggy bags are for).

WATERMELON

Foods with a high-water content, like watermelon (also cantaloupe and honeydew melon), fight fat because you get a lot of volume for few calories, explain nutritionists. And this melon is high in bloat-busting potassium, a mineral that can help you lose water weight as you fill up and not out when enjoying the superfruit. Watermelon is not only a summer superfood, you also can freeze it to enjoy the fruit year-round. Plus, watermelon seeds are growing in popularity and are another fat-burning food to add to your stay-lean diet repertoire.

Slim Down, Healthy Up Juices

Smoothies containing yogurt, milk, nuts, nutty butter, and other superfoods are good for you, but sometimes your body craves something cleaner, with fewer calories. Enter fresh fruit and fresh vegetable juice! As a child, I have fond memories of my mom using a hand juicer to make fresh orange juice on Sunday mornings, a day of a breakfast fit for royalty.

Instead of a fancy juicer, I ordered an inexpensive, low-tech citrus hand-juicer gadget, like mom's, for nostalgic reasons—and because reviews about pricey ones aren't, well, super. Plus, I'm not really a juicer fan. I prefer to eat whole fruits and vegetables to get all the fiber and nutrients, which some nutritionists and medical doctors believe is healthier than juicing away all the good stuff.

In my thirties, for instance, there was a popular hot tub facility in Palo Alto, California, that was my sanctuary to chill in between cramming for tests in grad school. Not only did each room boast a different tropical type of environment with foliage and Jacuzzi shapes complete with a sauna, but cold, fresh-squeezed orange juice (with all the pulp) was also sold in tall cups. It was heaven, and with the new juicer I plan to bring back the fond juice memories.

To help enhance the fat-fighting, healthful powers of juice-type smoothies, try these tips: Use raw fruits and vegetables. Raw foods contain live enzymes that are destroyed by cooking. Remember to wash all produce because of pesticides. But note, the skin of organic fruits is good for you so include the peel. Adding superfoods like nuts and seeds makes your skinny juice more filling, more healthful. Use honey or maple syrup, which are both rich in antioxidants, and these nature's sweeteners can help curb your sweet tooth so you won't be tempted to overindulge in unhealthy processed foods. Adding different spices can help boost your calorie-burning powers and provide extra flavor to your drink.

SLIMMING SUPERFOOD SMOOTHIES, SUPER TIPS

To enjoy the best smooth taste and texture:

- Add half a banana to any superfruit smoothie to make it extra creamy and thick. When you have more ripe bananas than you can use, peel them, cut in chunks, wrap in plastic wrap, and freeze.
- Add vanilla and other extracts for more flavor.
- Blend ice cubes into any smoothie to give it a milk-shake-like consistency and keep it chilled.
- Use real yogurt—forget the fat-free stuff—for a better taste and more protein. Plain or vanilla varieties are best.
- Add a spoonful of protein powder to up your protein intake, easily.

To boost your metabolism, enhance your smoothies in these ways:

- Use raw, whole superfruits and vegetables. Raw foods contain live enzymes that are destroyed in processed juices and cooked foods.

- Add nuts and seeds to get heart-healthy fats to help lower levels of "bad" LDL cholesterol.
- Use real maple syrup and honey—the premium, organic types— to sweeten smoothies naturally.
- Add spices and herbs such as cinnamon and basil for sweet and savory flavor.
- Stay clear of whole milk (except that occasionally using a small amount of organic half-and-half can be a treat if part of low-calorie ingredients).
- Smoothies ordered at ice cream shops can come with a lot of mystery ingredients that can pack on the pounds. If you have a choice, go homemade and be in control of slimming smoothies with fresh fruits, fresh vegetables, and all-natural flavorings and other ingredients.

LOSE UP TO SEVEN POUNDS ON THE TWO-DAY WEEKEND VEGETARIAN STONE-AGE DIET

Here is a jump-start diet plan. It is not intended to be used long-term. But you can use it one day per week or as needed after the first time which is two days, since it gives your body a vacation from too much overindulging in food on holidays or other special occasions that include rich and high-calorie fare.

Eating clean foods from a caveman, plant-based diet (berries, nuts, seeds, fish, and poultry that'll fill you) will help give your body a break— detoxing from sugar, meat, dairy, bad fats, and processed foods. Taking a mini–fast-food vacation can help you get fit and dump the muffin top, too.

This diet plan is adapted from umpteen minifasts I've created with the help of nutritionists. It also uses superfoods in the Oldways Mediterranean Diet Pyramid.

The Superfoods Stone-Age Diet Rules

- Do not go below one thousand calories. Keep in mind, olive oil contains 120 calories per tablespoon.
- Do not eat after 7 P.M. If you are hungry, you may eat a piece of fresh fruit with herbal tea.

- Health authorities advise you to drink seven to eight 8-ounce glasses of water daily. The amount depends on your size and weight, activity level, and where you live. (Seasons count, too; you may require more in hotter climate.)
- Consult with your health practitioner before starting this diet, or any new diet plan. Do not use if you're pregnant, nursing, or have diabetes.
- Take a daily multivitamin to help you get adequate nutrients.

Day 1

Before Breakfast
1 glass of hot water with fresh lemon

Breakfast
1 glass of bottled water with fresh lemon
1 apple or berries (no limit, but moderation is best)
Coffee or tea (1 cup black or white)

Snack
Herbal tea or 1 glass of fresh fruit-infused water

Lunch
Salad greens with olive oil, vinegar (your choice—apple cider or
  red wine), and spices/herbs to taste
Tea (1 cup black or white)
Fruit or berries
Herbal tea and/or bottled water

Dinner
1 handful nuts (walnuts or almonds)
1 cup cruciferous vegetables with fresh lemon (herbs and spices)
1 cup fresh melon chunks

Snack
Herbal tea

Day 2

Before Breakfast
6 ounces warm water with lemon

Breakfast
8 ounces coffee
1 bowl fresh fruit (mixed apples, berries) with handful of nuts, and sprinkled with seeds

Lunch
1 salad: Combine kale and spinach, 1 tablespoon sunflower seeds, strawberries, cranberries in moderation, 1 tablespoon olive oil mixed with balsamic vinegar to taste
1 apple

Snack
1 handful almonds, 3 dates
1 cup hot black or white tea

Dinner
1 cup cruciferous vegetables with lemon juice, herbs, and spices
½ cup quinoa or brown rice
1 small side dish of salad greens topped with tomatoes, seeds, drizzled with 1 tablespoon olive oil and a splash of balsamic vinegar

Super Wellness-Enhancing Autumn Apple-Pear Juice

Fall is my favorite season of the year. It's a time when food choices change and change is in the air. When I traveled to Montreal, Quebec, late one September, I made it a point to eat healthy, from airports to the hotel. This juice reminds me of the hotel breakfast menu, which offered an array of fresh fruits and fruit juices that made me feel like I was home, but in reality I was more than three thousand miles away from my comfort zone.

½ cup fresh, organic apple juice   ¼ banana

½ cup fresh pears, chopped   ½ cup ice cubes

Cinnamon stick

In a blender (use the smoothie button), blend juice, pears, banana, and ice until smooth. Pour into a mug. Garnish with cinnamon stick.

Makes 1 serving.

Now that you're on top of the aging game and eating superfoods without having to diet all the time, it's time to take our functional foods to another place. Yes, these foods can do much more than lower the risk of developing disease. My favorite superfoods can help you to cope with chronic ailments—all types. No kidding.

SUPER-IOR HEALING SUPERFOODS FOR THOUGHT

✓ Eating more skinny superfoods is the key to stoking your metabolism (calorie-burning power) and keeping lean.

✓ Grazing on fresh fruits and vegetables will fill you up, not out.

✓ Adding a balance of superfoods, including dairy, grains, poultry, nuts and seeds, and water, is the way to maintain good health and a healthy weight.

✓ Three big meals a day is twentieth-century thinking; enjoying five to six superfood minimeals is healthier for your mind and body, and you won't have hunger pangs.

SUPERFOOD CURES

Home Remedies from Your Kitchen

No disease that can be treated by diet should be treated with any other means.
—MAIMONIDES

After one trip to Canada, when I arrived home I was keen to the upheaval in the household. My second senior orange-and-white Brittany spaniel, Simon (a muse and mate for one fifth of my life) was distant—drifting away from me. A trip to the vet confirmed the news. Cognitive dysfunction syndrome, or aging of a dog's brain. After coping with painful Old Yeller-like ending days and nights, we lost the battle. My dog companion, of a breed known for its intelligence and sensitivity, exited the door of my household forever.

Grief-stricken, I ended up in the dermatologist's office. My eyelids were a light-brownish color. The physician's assistant asked me, "Have you been crying?" A tear trickled down my cheek. She took a photo of my brown eyes to show the doctor. The office music played "The

Sounds of Silence" by Simon and Garfunkel; the former being the inspiration for my late canine's name. The diagnosis: hyperpigmentation caused by aging and teardrops. There is no cure for heartbreak, but folk remedies can help suffering eyelids. I turned to lemons and used the juice diluted with water around my eyes. Within a few weeks, the brownish color was lighter. I used a lavender hypoallergenic eye shadow, and in time the brown color was fading, thanks to powers of nature's healing—and two superfoods—lemon and water.

SUPERFOOD HOME REMEDIES FOR 50 AILMENTS, A TO Z

I'll describe fifty health ailments from A to Z and provide reasons why there is a growing trend of do-it-yourself home remedies produced from foods in your pantry and kitchen cupboards, including the top 20 superfoods, their spin-off foods, and, to mix it up, other versatile superfoods. I added a dash of medical studies, sprinkled words of wisdom from nutritionists to medical doctors, and combined my own tried and true folk cures (some remedies are to be used inside and others outside the body) to make it a superfoods self-help list that may help you and yours.

1. ALLERGIES (COPE WITH ALLERGENS)

Autumn and spring are times when seasonal allergies can come into play. Culprits are longer than a cat's tail or an Australian shepherd's double-dense coat (achoo!), and they do include allergens, including pet dander, pollen, dust, and ragweed. Taking over-the-counter or prescription allergy pills can help a bit, but there is another natural antiallergy remedy to try.

What Superfoods Rx to Use: Quercetin-rich foods, such as apples, berries, and nuts, deliver this natural allergy fighter. Try adding fresh apple slices, berries, and a handful of nuts in your morning cereal or in a smoothie.

Why You'll Feel Supercharged: Quercetin is an antioxidant believed to act as a natural antihistamine. Instead of facing side effects of over-the-counter allergy pills, the superfoods remedy tastes good, and if you tend to have pesky allergy symptoms, such as sneezing, congestion, itchy eyes, and coughing, you'll feel better.

2. ANEMIA (GET MORE ENERGY)

Allergies are pesky, but anemia can be just as annoying. Eating a vegetarian diet, fad diets, or not eating enough and heavy menstrual periods in women during their reproductive years are some of the culprits. But anyone can be plagued by low iron, and it can bring on symptoms, including fatigue, pale skin, and lightheadedness.

What Superfoods Rx to Use: Eat foods rich in iron and vitamin B, such as a serving of shellfish (two or three times per week).

Why You'll Feel Supercharged: Eating iron-rich foods, such as shellfish, is just what doctors order. Anemia is more common in women during the childbearing years because of the monthly "curse," and vegetarians may lack the right amount of iron. Increasing your intake of vitamin B can help boost the iron lacking in your body and alleviating fatigue and other symptoms of not getting your iron on. Once you're back on track, symptoms linked to anemia should subside.

3. ANXIETY (TAKE CHILL TIME)

Frazzled nerves can be a challenge and often are linked to stress. If you feel on edge, with muscles tightened, you're probably anxious and ill at ease. Anxiety is a mind-body reaction and unsettling. However, you can take the control back and get into chill mode fast with the right superfoods and a blender. Superfoods such as berries, yogurt, and citrus can come to the rescue.

What Superfoods Rx to Use: Cranberry Shake: In a blender combine: ½ cup plain Greek yogurt; ¾ cup fresh cranberries or strawberries, whole; ¼ cup all-natural, fortified premium orange juice; ½ small banana, slices; ¼ cup organic half-and-half; 1 capful pure vanilla extract; honey to taste; 4–5 ice cubes; orange rind for topping garnish. Blend quickly until thick and smooth. Pour immediately into glass. Makes 1–2 servings.

Why You'll Feel Supercharged: Give credit to the banana, berries, and yogurt. The super thing is, fresh berries are an immunity-boosting stress buster because of their vitamin C content. The antistresser vitamin C can make a brain chemical, serotonin, that boosts those feel-good endorphins (like exercise can do). It also limits the production of adrenaline, which in turn helps people deal with stress.

Milk or yogurt can be nature's chill pill because of their calcium—a mineral that provides calming effects. Remember, having a cup of hot milk before bed is recommended to help you sleep. While you sip and spoon the creamy superfoods smoothie, its nutrients work to help you feel balanced and normal. Enjoy the chill!

4. ASTHMA (BREATHE MORE EASILY)

Anxiety is unsettling, just as is asthma, which is when the passageways in your lungs and trachea close up, making it difficult to breathe easily. Wheezing, coughing, and feeling a tightness in your chest can all be symptoms. Think of a fish out of water.

What Superfoods Rx to Use: Drink seven to eight 8-ounce glasses of water daily. Add one serving of tomatoes in your diet regime, whether it's a serving of juice, a sliced tomato, or marinara sauce.

Why You'll Feel Supercharged: Keeping hydrated with water (and water-dense fruits and vegetables like berries and tomatoes) can help keep the airways lubricated and detoxified against allergens (such as smoke and pet dander), which could keep an asthma attack at bay. It's the lycopene in tomatoes that may lessen the effects of exercise-induced asthma, according to past medical research on people who suffer from asthma, including their triggers for the condition and what remedies can help curb attacks.

5. AUTOIMMUNE DISORDERS (TAKE BACK CONTROL)

Anxiety can affect all of us sometime during our lifetime, whether it's a quick anxious moment while on an airplane with rough air or something linked to hormonal challenges. But autoimmune disorders (rheumatoid arthritis to lupus and many in-between) occur when the immune system works against itself. By strengthening immunity, you can help to ward off or lessen its effects or flare-ups.

What Superfoods Rx to Use: Eat sea vegetables, such as dulse or nori, a few times per week. Add them to salads, soups, stews, or even a savory smoothie.

Why You'll Feel Supercharged: Red-algae ocean veggies, such as dulse and nori, but also blue-green algae (like spirulina), help deter viruses that affect the immune system, thanks to their antiviral properties. That means their antioxidants, vitamins, and minerals help to bolster immunity. Past research has shown a link to eating sea vegetables and a healthier immune system, and some medical doctors definitely give them a thumbs-up as a superfood that makes it to the superfoods list.

6. THE BLUES (SAVOR HAPPY FOODS)

An asthma attack is nothing to take lightly, nor is a bout of the blues (short-term sadness or feeling in a slump). However, it's not uncommon to feel a bit down during hectic holidays or sometimes without rhyme or reason. One time when feeling misery, as an inquisitive one, down or up, I took an online test to find out if I was coping with depression or the blues. The answer was the latter. Somewhat relieved that my blues would pass, I turned to the superfoods cure.

What Superfoods Rx to Use: Try eating brazil nuts and/or sunflower seeds (chased by a square of dark chocolate). Repeat twice a day.

Why You'll Feel Supercharged: Eating selenium-rich foods, such as brazil nuts and sunflower seeds, can spike blood selenium levels, which can help boost your mood. Plus, chocolate contains a brain chemical called serotonin that can make you feel happier and improve brainpower and memory. When your serotonin level is low, you can feel the winter or summertime blues. Recipe: Heat 12 ounces dark chocolate (chips or a bar) in the microwave for a minute or until melted. Stir in 1/4 cup seeds and 3 nuts, chopped. Spread into a rectangle shape on a parchment-lined cookie sheet. Place chocolate in the freezer for approximately 20 minutes or until firm. Remove the chocolate and break into peanut-brittle-type pieces. Put into an airtight container. The chocolate nut-seed bark lasts up to two weeks.

7. BRAIN FOG (FEEL MORE ALERT!)

Feeling the blues usually goes away, as can a lack of mental alertness. If you use your brainpower on the job or at play and/or relaxation, you might later experience a fuzziness, unclear thinking, and indecisiveness, which can be like being in a fog! There are different reasons why brain fog happens, including side effects of cholesterol medications, sleep deprivation, and unexpected life changes and challenges. Whatever the cause of you not being well off, brain foods can help you to think sharper.

What Superfoods Rx to Use: Eat one serving of walnuts at least a few times per week.

Why You'll Feel Supercharged: Foods that are rich in omega-3 fatty acids, including walnuts, can help fight off fuzzy thinking. Getting the right amount of good fat, like that found in nuts, can help keep brain chemicals called neurotransmitters balanced and functioning the way they normally do, so you feel clear-headed.

8. CANKER SORES (HEAL THE PAIN)

Coping with fuzzy thoughts is a problem that can be fixed quickly, but if a canker sore pays you a visit, its stay may linger longer than you'd want it to. If you'd ever had one of these little red lesions inside your mouth (often on the inner cheek), it's normal to seek out any remedy to soothe the hurt. The cause can be stress, spicy foods, a trauma, or even a chemical in toothpaste. But the good news is there is something that can speed up the healing process.

What Superfoods Rx to Use: There are a few remedies that can be combined to do the job. Try sea salt and warm water rinses 3 to 4 times daily. Suck on ice cubes. Eat cool, creamy plain Greek yogurt and a bit of Manuka honey. Also, drinking chamomile tea as needed can calm the pain.

Why You'll Feel Supercharged: While some over-the-counter medications can numb the pain, dental pastes prescribed by your dentist can help, too, by forming a seal over the sore. However, the superfoods recommended do not have side effects and can be effective, too. In a nutshell, the salt water is an anti-inflammatory with antibacterial benefits. Ice can chill the burn and ache of the sore. Yogurt and honey feel good to eat when you're hungry, and they also boast anti-inflammatory and antibacterial perks like salt water as well as calming chamomile. The average course of time for a canker sore to heal can be ten to fourteen days. If you follow the superfoods recipe, within three days you'll be on the road to recovery.

9. CLOGGED ARTERIES (CLEAN THE PLAQUE)

Hardening of the arteries isn't something young people think about, but plaque buildup can affect your heart health as you age. Keeping heart-healthy becomes more of a priority in the senior and elderly years and is key to living a longer, healthier life. So, can superfoods help keep our arteries running smoothly?

What Superfoods Rx to Use: Drink an 8-ounce glass of grape juice and/or pomegranate juice (without added sugar) every day.

Why You'll Feel Supercharged: Stacks of research have shown grape juice and pomegranate juice can help the cells in our body suffer less damage from physical stress, such as high blood pressure. The antioxidant-rich fruit juice can ward off hardening of the arteries; keeping the blood flowing and circulation moving is recommended before you're prescribed blood thinners, which come with a mixed bag of side effects. For more information, check out the American Heart Association's website on heart health and cholesterol.

10. COLDS AND FLU (AVOID THE VIRUS)

Keeping a watch on cholesterol is important as an adult, and staving off colds and the flu (especially with different strains) is not to be ignored, either. The ancient remedy called chicken soup, praised by holistic medical proponents and food historians, goes back, way back in time before your mother and her mother hit the kitchen to make a batch of the homemade cure. As the legend goes, in 60 A.D., a surgeon to the Roman emperor Nero documented the superfood to other doctors by touting chicken soup to be a food and medicine.[1]

What Superfoods Rx to Use: Savor a bowl of hot chicken soup (preferably homemade with vegetables) once or twice daily. Repeat as needed.

Why You'll Feel Supercharged: Chicken soup, with protein and calming vitamin B vitamins from poultry and antioxidants in onions and other vegetables (e.g., carrots, tomatoes) can help with congestion and enhance the immune system back to health. The hot liquid can help, too, by soothing aches and pains and by coating a sore throat.

The Tale of Chicken Soup

Food historians will share the tale of a twelfth-century doctor, Moses Maimonides, who gave credit to the healing powers of chicken soup as a super remedy. As the legend goes, a military leader was desperate to help battle his son's asthma. The doctor's orders weren't a medical treatment but good, old-fashioned chicken soup.

It's been said that our great-grandmothers made chicken soup from ingredients on a farm. Our grandmas put together chicken soup from a vegetable garden. Our moms used a canned or boxed soup.

And today, in the twenty-first century, many younger generations, to the baby boomers, like me, are going back to nature and incorporating farm-to-table vegetables as well as finding out the source of their chicken (cage free, grass fed, and organic) for the best chicken soup.

11. CONSTIPATION (GET SUPER REGULAR)

When I was a graduate student, a regular bathroom schedule wasn't part of my busy curriculum. I remember that my mate's mother, a health-oriented woman in her early fifties, shared her secret to staying regular. "Each morning I drink a cup of hot water and lemon juice." Stubborn as I was, I didn't follow the regime and was uncomfortable by the day's end. I ended up at the office of a stomach doctor, who wrote down on a prescription pad: "More water, more fiber." In retrospect, I should have listened to the good doctor and the wise woman, who ended up living a full and healthy life to her octogenarian years.

What Superfoods Rx to Use: Heat 12 ounces of bottled water and add 2 tablespoons of fresh lemon juice. Also, drink seven to eight 8-ounce glasses of water every day. An apple a day can also help keep you regular.

Why You'll Feel Supercharged: Water and lemon keep constipation at bay. The fiber in lemons is good for your digestion, and it can help detoxify your body, too. Also, I didn't need to go to college to discover black tea (with its caffeine content) with lemon can help get things moving along, too. The dietary fiber in apples can be helpful, too, to keep your system regular.

Taking Care of Business on the Road and Off

When traveling, getting off the regularity track is almost par for the course. It may be due to the irregular schedule of being sedentary on planes and trains or eating a different diet. But I've learned how to take back the control to keep regular. One trip to Seattle, I went on a trek through Pike Place Market to find dried prunes. This seemed to me like an easy find, but it was not. Vendors wanted to sell me a huge bag of the dried fruit, not a small bag, which is all I needed to be able to let nature take its course. I ended up in a little tea shop and sat at the counter. I explained my plight to the counter girl, but she looked at me like I was from another planet. She served me a complimentary cup of tea and listened to me complain about Day 4 of not making a visit to the bathroom. I got no tips of what type of tea to sip and savor, so I left still clueless. Once home, after a cup of coffee in the afternoon to battle jet lag, I was relieved and back to normal.

The next trip, I came with my arsenal of go-to foods. I always had bottled water in hand and a small bag of dried prunes in my purse paired with fresh green apples. When laid over at airports or train stations, I was drinking chamomile tea or coffee. And breakfast, lunch, and dinner always included a vegetable-stocked salad. On the next trip to

Victoria, British Columbia, I used this recipe, and in the morning, it was like I was at home; comfort and regularity paid me a welcome visit.

Apple, Kale and Honey Juice

A green drink is not my fantasy beverage, perhaps because sipping the dark-green-colored goo isn't easy on the eyes. But, like inching my way into a chilly swimming pool, combining apples and kale with a bit of spice and honey is something that works well, and no cold feet. I've seen a few Hallmark Channel films where characters whip up a green concoction and offer it to their guests—who are anything but thrilled to drink it. But my lighter-green version of a healthful green drink with sweet superfoods may be just the trick to blend up for you, and to serve to your friends and family, too.

*2 medium Fuji or
  Honeycrisp organic
  apples, quartered,
  cored, and seeded
¼ cup kale, washed,
  chopped*

*½ teaspoon cinnamon
1 teaspoon raw honey
Fresh lemon juice, to
  taste*

Combine apples and kale in a juicer, process the ingredients. Add cinnamon, honey, and lemon.

Makes 1 serving.

12. COUGH (STOP THE TICKLE)

Enjoying the ease of regularity is essential to good health and well-being and even boosts your energy levels and mood. However, if you develop a cough, perhaps after a cold, or worse, a bout of bronchitis, you won't be feeling on the top of your game, either. Can a superfood help tame the tickle in your throat and stop the hacking? If your cough is moderate, superfoods can come to the rescue.

What Superfoods Rx to Use: Use 2 tablespoons of fresh lemon juice in a cup of chamomile tea. Add honey to taste. Repeat as needed.

Why You'll Feel Supercharged: Citrus fruit, much like tea and honey, contains anti-inflammatory and antibacterial properties. Instead of turning to prescription antibiotics or cough drops, this superfood remedy will coat your throat as well as work on inflammation. Pairing these superfoods may help cure the cough. But note, if your cough is severe or doesn't subside in a few days, consult with your health practitioner.

13. DEHYDRATION (FUEL IT UP)

Staying hydrated while healing from a cold is key, but drinking water is essential for overall good health and well-being. If you are not drinking enough fluids, symptoms may pay you a visit. Headaches, muscle cramps, lightheadedness, and constipation are just a few of the challenges that come with not getting an adequate amount of H_2O.

What Superfoods Rx to Use: Drink seven to eight 8-ounce glasses of water per day. If it's a hot climate or if you've been exercising, you may need more.

Why You'll Feel Supercharged: Getting enough water provides a myriad of healing powers. You'll feel energized, be more regular, and enjoy a healthy facial glow. Water is a superfood, and we cannot survive without it. It is much healthier than sugary drinks, diet sodas, or fruit juices with added sugar. Herbal teas, however, can help you stay hydrated like plain water.

14. DENTAL CAVITIES (HALT THE HOLES)

Drinking water to avoid dehydration is an easier task than avoiding dental caries. Cavities or decay are caused by bacteria and can lead to worse dental woes, like fillings, crowns, root canals, and tooth loss. But there is an arsenal you can create to lessen the likelihood of tooth problems. Enter the right foods to snack on or eat during meals.

What Superfoods Rx to Use: Eat a cup of plain yogurt a day and/or a serving of cheese.

Why You'll Feel Supercharged: Research suggests that eating wholesome calcium-containing foods, like yogurt and cheese, instead of sugary and starchy foods, may be helpful in the prevention of dental cavities. The calcium in cheese and yogurt contains antimicrobial properties, and it may be useful in coating and strengthening teeth.

15. DEPRESSION (GOOD RIDDANCE, DESPAIR)

Dental caries are not as common in the twenty-first century if good dental hygiene is practiced, but feeling blue or down is a malady that has been timeless, probably from caveman days to medieval times to the present day. If it's a mild bout of feeling depressed which can include feeling fatigue, not interested in normal activities, it may be due to a temporary situation, such as job loss or money challenges. Using your coping skills and exercise can be helpful, as might a healthy diet full of superfoods. No time for unhealthy empty nutrition foods. But which one can boost your mood and help you to snap out of it and move on with a mind-body positive movement-forward attitude?

What Superfoods Rx to Use: Eat 3 servings of fresh fruit each day paired with at least two cups of tea.

Why You'll Feel Supercharged: Fruit, such as crunchy apples, will help defrazzle your nerves and ease the anxiety and stress that often can spawn a bout of depression. Drinking tea will keep you feeling energized, as will fresh fruit. This, in return, will help give you an incentive to get a move on and exercise. Studies show exercise does boost feel-good hormones like endorphins and will help you to battle that down feeling and lift up your spirits.

16. DIARRHEA (STOP BATHROOM RUNS)

Feeling down is a drag, but having to go to the bathroom more rather than less can be downright depressing! This problem can be caused by eating food that doesn't agree with you, taking a course of antibiotics, the stomach flu, and other reasons. Rather than turn to over-the-counter medication, there are superfoods that can come to the rescue.

What Superfoods Rx to Use: Eat ½ ounce of dried blueberries twice per day. Repeat as needed. Add 6 ounces of plain Greek yogurt twice a day.

Why You'll Feel Supercharged: This remedy is rich in anthocyanosides, which can help destroy bad bacteria, so it may help stop the urge to go. Yogurt is touted to help calm and normalize a volatile digestive problem, including a bout of the runs. Its probiotics are the gems that give it its antibacterial action, which can help stop the "go" and put your stomach functions back in normal working order for you.

17. DIZZINESS (STEADY YOUR GROUNDING)

Spending too much time in the bathroom is not fun, nor is feeling lightheaded and dizzy. There are many causes of dizziness, but common causes are not eating and dehydration. During my Victoria, British Columbia, adventure, I booked back-to-back adventures, including visiting the wharf to find a seal, but I forgot to drink water. On the wharf, I felt a bit lightheaded and sat down on a bench to feel grounded. I wasn't drinking water! After I drank a 12-ounce bottled water, the undesirable symptoms of feeling out of balance were gone and did not return. From that day on, I make a point to eat and to drink water and to not forget, no matter how busy I am. That said, are you wondering what superfood to go to for help to keep balanced?

What Superfoods Rx to Use: Every day, eat a nutrient-dense diet full of a balance of superfoods, including fruits, vegetables, protein, dairy, and most importantly, water, water, water.

Why You'll Feel Supercharged: Your body needs adequate nourishment, as does your brain, which is approximately 75 percent water. If you deprive yourself of superfoods, including adequate water intake, it isn't unheard of to feel a bit unsteady. To stave off lightheadedness and stay grounded, water intake is essential.

Earwax and the Superfood Cure

Speaking of dizziness, did you know earwax, known as cerumen, can be a pain in the inner ear that can ultimately affect your balance, too? Impacted earwax can cause a feeling of fullness in ears, coughing, and even earaches.

As a devout swimmer, I've experienced flare-ups of swimmer's ear, or otitis externa, a painful condition that has cleared up with prescription eardrops. But earwax (which is normal and actually protects our ears) hadn't been a problem until it paid me an unwelcome visit that I'll never forget . . .

One day at a regular doctor's checkup, I asked my general practitioner to take a look inside my ears. He said they were impacted with earwax. Blame it on the cotton swabs I used at a pool. Doctor's orders were simple. Use an at-home self-care kit of earwax softener and use a bulb to flush with water after. Easy enough, right? Wrong. I asked without knowledge of impacted earwax to have my ears flushed instead of using earwax-softener drops. Multiple water ear flushings later at the doctor's office, I got a rude awakening. If the earwax is too hard and the water temperature is too cold or hot, dizziness can happen. As my world was spinning, nausea set in. (The procedure affects your inner ear and equilibrium.) I left the office disoriented, with wax in my Dumbo-like ears.

Five days later, with fantasies of severing my ear like Van Gogh, I made an appointment to see an ear, nose, and throat specialist. These days, it's common to have earwax removed by a microsuction machine to vacuum out earwax. No messy irrigation. It is easy, fast, and painless. I survived the ear incident. I learned two lessons. One, do not use cotton swabs except to clean the outer ear. Two, do flush your ears with body-temperature superfood water once a week in the shower. And you'll be able to keep both ears.

18. FIBROMYALGIA (LOSE THE ACHES)

An ear incident is not a fun event, nor are aches and pains due to inflamed nerves. Years ago, fibromyalgia was not acknowledged by doctors, but now we know it's a real problem and not all in the head. People with fibromyalgia suffer from chronic pain, stiffness, and tenderness in their muscles and related soft tissues. There are eighteen tender checkpoints in the body used to diagnose this condition, but even if you do not have pain in each one, it still doesn't mean you're not suffering.

What Superfoods Rx to Use: Eat one serving of cranberries (fresh or dried) every day as needed.

Why You'll Feel Supercharged: Vitamin C–rich berries can work wonders for aches and pains. The antioxidant supervitamin can help make collagen, a protein that builds and repairs cartilage and muscles. It also can help fight inflammation. Once you feel less or no pain, you're more apt to exercise, which triggers the brain's release of natural pain-killing compounds, like endorphins. Also, you'll boost the feel-good brain chemical serotonin (found in superfoods like dark chocolate). This, in turn, can help you to chill, and when you're calm, your pain can be less and your muscles more relaxed.

19. FOOD POISONING (PRACTICE EATING SAFETY)

Tight muscles are a challenge, but getting sick from food is something we all would like to dodge. There is a natural, preventative way to beat the battle of spoiled food before it hits your tummy. Sometimes, you don't have a say about something you've eaten or drunk and you're blindsided by bacteria. One night, I was at a movie theatre and I ordered a coffee latte. Twenty minutes later, my stomach began to gurgle. I was in the bathroom during the entire film. I blamed my demise on the coffee. The girl at the coffee counter fessed up, "Maybe it was the soap residue on the dirty coffee decanter."

What Superfoods Rx to Use: Try putting 2 teaspoons of apple cider vinegar in a 12-ounce bottled water.

Why You'll Feel Supercharged: Vinegar is known to have antibacterial compounds in it. These mighty workers can help stave off bacteria found on food, such as at picnics or even a cruise. If you drink a vinegar cocktail before you indulge, it may be just what you need to stay well and avoid any upset stomach that can wreak havoc on your plans and body.

20. GINGIVITIS (BABY THOSE GUMS)

Food poisoning comes on fast, whereas inflammation of the gums in the mouth can occur over time, due to neglect, stress, hormones, and genetics. The good news is that red and swollen gums can be a temporary and reversible ailment.

What Superfoods Rx to Use: Eat 6 ounces of plain Greek yogurt with a bit of raw honey each day, chased with an 8-ounce glass of orange juice fortified with calcium and vitamin D. Also, drink seven to eight 8-ounce glasses of water per day.

Why You'll Feel Supercharged: Calcium-rich foods like Greek yogurt can build up your immune system and help strengthen your teeth. By turning to plain yogurt, you'll bypass added sugars in flavored yogurts. Research has shown the power of superfood yogurt against gingivitis in middle-aged men and women. People who ate less yogurt, with its friendly bacteria, had more advanced gum disease than those who consumed the superfood, according to the scientists, who give credit to the active cultures in yogurt that protect against gingivitis.

Honey is also an excellent home remedy for gingivitis because of its anti-inflammatory and antibacterial properties. The vitamin C–rich citrus is a known gingivitis fighter that goes back to the days of sailors at sea who beat gum disease. And, of course, brushing your teeth twice a day and flossing will help keep gingivitis at bay.

21. HEADACHES (STOP THE THROBBING)

Sore gums are a headache, so to speak, but a real headache can also be a pain. Migraines are terrible, but tension headaches are the most common type (up to 90 percent), according to headache experts at the National Headache Foundation.

What Superfoods Rx to Use: Opt for two to three servings per week of vitamin B–rich superfoods like lean, organic poultry (chicken and turkey).

Why You'll Feel Supercharged: Incorporating chicken or turkey into your diet may help boost levels of serotonin, a brain chemical that can lower headache pain. Plus, vitamin B_{12} may help the brain to function better, lessening an oncoming headache, which is often linked to stress.

22. HEARTBURN (SOOTHE THE BURN)

You likely have endured a tension headache sometime in your life, not unlike a bout of heartburn on occasion. Heartburn is acid indigestion or gastroesophageal reflux disease (GERD). It happens when stomach acid flows back up your esophagus, the tube that carries food to your stomach. Images of the characters in the foodie lovers' film *Julie & Julia* come to mind, as they reach for antacids after a fatty dish, which we probably are all guilty of doing, especially during the holidays, whether we cooked it or someone else did the deed with unwitting damage.

Too much tomato sauce on pasta or pizza or just plain overindulgence (rarely do I do that anymore because heartburn isn't worth it) are my personal demons. So if I, like perhaps you, too, may fall victim to heartburn through fault of my own or not, I want immediate relief.

What Superfoods Rx to Use: Eat ½ cup plain Greek yogurt. Repeat once or twice a day as needed.

Why You'll Feel Supercharged: The cool yogurt may get rid of the burn for a variety of reasons. It contains good bacteria for the digestive tract. The protein-rich food may help prevent acid reflux during digestion (that's if you eat if before the damage is done). Yogurt also may help strengthen muscles in the lower esophagus. And last, but certainly not to be least, creamy yogurt can help lessen inflammation or gas in the intestine, and therefore the burning chest pain and or pressure in the neck and throat is not as bothersome. Yogurt, then, can make that burning sensation subside, much like an over-the-counter heartburn medication can do.

23. HERPES (HEAL THE BLISTERS)

A temporary bout of heartburn will pass, as will a herpes flare-up. Herpes is a viral infection that can be caused by herpes simplex virus 1 (cold sores) or herpes simplex virus 2 (genital herpes). Coping with an outbreak can be painful, both physically and emotionally. If you have dealt with herpes, you may wonder, "Is there a superfood that can help prevent it from happening?" After all, getting little red bumps and blisters is not only an inconvenience, but it can occur at times when it's the last thing you want during an important event.

What Superfoods Rx to Use: Try eating 1 serving of seaweed three times per week.

Why You'll Feel Supercharged: Past research, including findings at the Naval Biosciences Laboratory at the University of California, Berkeley, has shown that the herpes virus may be halted by eating seaweed—especially from the red-algae family. In fact, in a lab study, seaweed extracts showed that they inhibited herpes quickly.

24. HIGH BLOOD PRESSURE (CONTROL THE NUMBERS)

Herpes is not life threatening, but high blood pressure numbers can be risky business. Simply put, blood pressure consists of two forces. When taking a blood pressure reading, the top number, the systolic pressure, describes the pressure of your blood in your arteries when your heart contracts, and the bottom number, the diastolic pressure, describes the blood pressure between heartbeats. Stress can increase your readings, as well as what you eat. The good news is, if you add more superfoods to your diet and lose processed sugary and high-sodium food, you may be able to get your blood pressure down to normal at 120 over 80 or lower.

What Superfoods Rx to Use: Each day, include two to three servings of water-dense fruits in your diet. Try melons and berries. A fresh fruit smoothie with fresh water ice cubes is ideal.

Why You'll Feel Supercharged: Nutrient-dense fruit, such as fresh watermelon and strawberries, can help counteract sodium in your body, and the potassium can help blood pressure numbers to be normal. Also, getting regular exercise, destressing, and maintaining an ideal weight will help, too.

25. INFECTIONS (BOOST YOUR IMMUNITY)

High blood pressure is more common with aging, but a bacterial infection can affect us at any age. Some surprising superfoods may be super infection fighters that you may want to incorporate in your diet. Infections, from head to toe, are nothing to take lightly, and if a superfood can strengthen your immune system, you may be able to dodge being affected by bacteria and their consequences.

What Superfoods Rx to Use: Use maple syrup in your smoothies, top oatmeal with it, and drizzle it over whole-grain French toast at least three times per week.

Why You'll Feel Supercharged: Plenty of research in eastern Canada points to maple syrup and its abilities to fight different types of infections. The Federation of Quebec Maple Syrup Producers claims maple syrup contains more than one hundred bioactive compounds, and many of these may be among nature's defenses against bacteria. One study conducted at Canada's McGill University and published in the journal *Applied and Environmental Microbiology* discovered that an extract of maple syrup can combat bacteria that cause infections, including E. coli and urinary tract infections. In fact, it may even slash the use of prescription antibiotics that come with side effects.[2]

26. INSOMNIA (GET GOOD SLEEP)

Coping with infections can be draining, but not getting adequate shut-eye can turn your world upside down. Sleep deprivation can make you cranky and unable to perform your best at work and play, as well as tax your body and well-being. If you're trying to get a good night's sleep, eating enough superfoods—the right ones—may be your natural nightcap.

What Super Rx to Use: Dish up a serving of plain Greek yogurt, drizzle a bit of raw honey on top, and mix.

Why You'll Feel Supercharged: Greek yogurt is rich in magnesium and calcium. These minerals act as natural tranquilizers in your body and can help calm you to promote restful sleep.

27. IRRITABLE BOWEL SYNDROME (TEND TO PLUMBING)

Not getting essential shut-eye is unhealthy since sleep helps to rejuvenate the body, and an abnormal digestive system routine also can wreak havoc on your gut. When I fell victim to crazy crash diets (diet soda and bubble gum), I met irritable bowel syndrome—a pesky and painful visitor I will never forget.

What Super Rx to Use: Eat a fiber-rich apple each day and drink seven to eight 8-ounce glasses of water each day. Also, add 6 ounces of plain Greek yogurt to your daily diet regime.

Why You'll Feel Supercharged: Pairing the dietary fiber found in apples with water is key to keeping regular. Research shows water can help your digestive system to stay on course, like a sink with a drain that is kept unclogged. Plus, consuming Greek yogurt, which is rich in probiotics (live bacteria called active cultures), can help keep your digestive tract healthier, restore balance, and keep your system running smoothly. It's the probiotics in yogurt that stave off the "bad" bacteria. Also, keep in mind, irritable bowel syndrome results from a body-mind connection. So, staying physical will help keep you more centered and less stressed—the essentials of keeping your bowels calm and letting you enjoy a sense of normalcy.

28. JET LAG (FEEL THE NORMAL)

Speaking of going (or not) and travel, jet lag is something we all may endure if our schedule gets a shake-up due to long hours on a plane and lack of sleep. It's a pesky problem, wherein you can feel sluggish teamed with brain fog. So, is there anything you can do that is healthful, natural, and will give you a boost of energy?

What Superfoods Rx to Use: Drink a glass of fresh lemon-infused water paired with a handful of nuts.

Why You'll Feel Supercharged: Water can help provide instant energy, and fresh lemon or orange juice can give you a boost of nature's carbohydrates, which can also be energizing. Protein-rich nuts, much like water and fruit, can boost your energy levels, thanks to their nutrients of magnesium and selenium. If you ever wonder why flight attendants serve nuts on a plane, this could be the reason.

29. KIDNEY STONES (STOP ANY BLOCKAGE)

A friend of mine developed painful kidney stones when he was in his forties. The doctors suspected it could have been linked to low fluid intake. I recall he told me of the ordeal to get rid of those painful stones. An appointment was made to blast the stones with shock waves in a bathtub-type setting, called lithotripsy. There had to be a more traditional, back-to-nature way to prevent kidney stones, right?

What Superfoods Rx to Use: Drink 1 glass of water with fresh lemon juice every morning. Also, do keep hydrated with seven to eight 8-ounce glasses of water every day.

Why You'll Feel Supercharged: Homemade lemonade boasts citrates, which are part of citric acid. The theory is that citric acid stops calcium-based stones from forming. It is known by medical doctors that lemon can and does help detoxify your body.

30. LACKLUSTER LIBIDO (BOOST SEX DRIVE)

Kidney stones can be very painful, but if we can prevent them or get rid of them, we don't have to deal with the pain at all, but our sex drive is something that can wax and wane throughout our lives, for a variety of reasons. I recall one doctor who believes he can tell if a patient is healthy by observing three things: skin texture, energy level, and if an individual has their libido intact. If all of these are good, it is a good sign. Of course there is more to good health than this simple test, but in a pinch it seems to make sense, despite the consequences of Eve taking the first bite of an apple in the garden.

What Superfoods Rx to Use: Consume one apple (preferably organic) every day, and leave the skin on, but be sure to rinse it with water first to get rid of any potential pesticide residue.

Why You'll Feel Supercharged: Low-fat, fiber-rich apples are believed to enhance the sex drive in both women and men for many reasons. Not only can the fruit help keep you regular, which gives you more energy, but due to its abundance of minerals and vitamins, it also can help boost your overall health and well-being. Apples are low in calories, so the fruit can help you maintain an ideal weight, which can also give you an edge in the romance department because you'll feel better in both mind and body.

31. LOVESICKNESS (FILL THE VOID)

From a sluggish sex drive, feeling low because you lose a loved one can be more of a challenge. After living life for many decades, I admit to coping with lovesickness more than libidinal woes. Loving and losing a loved one is challenging. When loss hits us, it's not uncommon to also lose our appetite. But superfoods can help you get through this roller coaster time of emotions.

What Superfoods Rx to Use: Drink seven to eight 8-ounce glasses of water each day. Add fresh superfruits and vegetables. Take a multivitamin supplement.

Why You'll Feel Supercharged: If you don't drink water, you'll get dehydrated and be welcomed by a host of health ailments. So, go ahead. Drink water (flavor it up with sliced lemon or lime), and savor your favorite tea, too. We know plant-based vegan diets can be healthful due to their abundance of nutrients. So, during times when your appetite is lacking, nibble on fresh fruit (including slices of apples and whole berries) and enjoy your favorite vegetables (crucifers and sweet potatoes). Not only will you be feeding your body, but you'll also be nourishing your mind and spirit. Does food help heal a broken heart? Well, not technically, but it will get you through the stages of grief and help to keep you well.

32. MORNING SICKNESS (CALM YOUR TUMMY)

Feeling queasy due to pregnancy is a completely different ache from lovesickness, but it causes its own kind of discomfort for some women. Nausea that waxes and wanes is not fun, and saltine crackers and coping with it knowing the queasy feeling will pass (much like sea sickness) can work. But there is a superfood (or two) that can be helpful to find a new normalcy during the swells of the body.

What Superfoods Rx to Use: Eat 6 ounces of vanilla Greek yogurt or plain yogurt drizzled with raw honey. Repeat twice a day.

Why You'll Feel Supercharged: Cool, creamy yogurt can be soothing to the upset digestive system, whether it's due to pregnancy, motion sickness, or antibiotics, which can cause borderline nausea. Vanilla is known to be a calming spice, whereas honey contains antibacterial compounds and can soothe that queasy feeling in the tummy. But note, do not give honey to an infant.

33. MUSCLE PAIN (LOOSEN THE TIGHTNESS)

Morning sickness isn't fun, but muscle aches and pains can seem worse if you're the one with an arm or leg that hurts. Age can play a role, but not always. When I was in my twenties, I swam one hundred laps of breaststroke. The next day, I paid the price with my rib cage aching (on a 1 to 10 scale, it was a 20). Time healed the muscle pain, but you may discover as you grow older that it may take longer to heal the pain. Common sense is key, including warming up before exercise and lifting heavy objects the right way, from your legs not your back, but sometimes muscle pain occurs without being mindful. For instance, allowing my Australian shepherd, Skyler, to walk me while walking him and vacuuming with a new, heavy vacuum cleaner certainly helped an unwelcome muscle strain. So, what to do?

What Superfoods Rx to Use: Every one or two hours, apply an ice pack on the body area affected with aches. Pair with one glass of fruit juice, such as cherry or watermelon.

Why You'll Feel Supercharged: Water and cold, cold ice can help lessen inflammation. Once the inflamed muscles are treated, the pain usually subsides. Cherries added to your superfoods list can help block inflammation and halt pain enzymes, much like over-the-counter pain medications. Research shows that either drinking cherry juice or eating a bowl of cherries, which contain antioxidants, can help reduce pain. Also, don't forget the healing power of watermelon juice. It may help soothe muscle soreness after a workout thanks to the substance citrulline, which may relax blood vessels, as reported in the *Journal of Agriculture and Food Chemistry*.[3]

34. PANIC ATTACK (FACE THE MONSTERS)

Muscle strains are challenging, but when anxiety hits, ending up in a full-blown panic attack, it's super scary. Think of the agoraphobic character in the film *Copycat* when she ends up with her caretaker giving her a paper bag for hyperventilating. In my lifetime, I've experienced and lived to share the tales of coping with panic attacks, often spawned by stress, and even other culprits can be to blame. Before and during an anxiety attack, you can feel a loss of control. Symptoms such as lightheadedness, tense muscles, and a racing heart can all be part of it. Think how you'd react to severe rough air on an airplane or a major earthquake, and that is how an attack can sneak up on you and—*BAM!*—make you feel spooked.

What Superfoods Rx to Use: Try drinking a full 12-ounce bottle of water; sip it all until it's gone. Also, sip herbal tea (hot or iced) throughout the day.

Why You'll Feel Supercharged: Water can be a godsend if an anxiety attack pays you a visit, whether you're up in the air or on the ground. If you don't stay hydrated, it can affect your blood flow. Muscles may tense up, stress sets in, and it can lead to lightheadedness. This, in turn, can lead to anxiety. So, no matter where you are, whether it be the dentist or doctor's office, onboard a plane, or at home working, make it a point to have water nearby to sip and savor and stave off any type of anxiety.

35. PLAQUE/TARTAR (LOSE THE GUNK)

Panic can be big trouble, but it usually passes, whereas plaque (the sticky stuff that builds up on your teeth within twenty-four hours or less after brushing) is an unwelcome visitor that continues to try and ruin your dental health routine. Worse, if you allow plaque to develop, it can turn into tartar (the calcium deposits that are brownish and only can be scraped off by dental pros. So, is there a superfood that can help you protect against plaque?

What Superfoods Rx to Use: Eat a square of cheese three or four times per week, especially as a snack.

Why You'll Feel Supercharged: Say hello again to cheese. It helps in the production of alkaline saliva that can neutralize the acid in plaque. It can aid in creating a protective layer around your teeth. Also, cheese contains calcium and phosphorus, which can help remineralize your teeth.

Past research notes that cheese (without added sugar) may help to prevent dental cavities in children by boosting calcium and phosphorus, keeping dental plaque at bay.

36. POISON OAK/IVY (SOOTHE THE ITCH)

Most of us have had dental hygienists scrape off tartar, but perhaps fewer of us have had to endure the painful itching of poison oak or poison ivy, yet most humans are not immune to the scourge of the rash from these plants. Imagine itchy skin, red bumps, and blisters that can spread easily.

What Superfoods Rx to Use: Fill a cloth bag or sachet with dry rolled oats. Tie the bag and put it in a bowl or tub of water. Then place the wet bag on the affected area for 15 minutes. Repeat as needed. Also, for even quicker relief, you may try placing cool, plain yogurt on the skin.

Why You'll Feel Supercharged: Getting relief from the stinging and itchiness that comes with a bout of skin rashes like poison oak or poison ivy is a good thing. If you've ever suffered from the symptoms, you'll understand that you want the itchiness to stop.

37. PROSTATE PROBLEMS (NIBBLE FOR NORMALCY)

Skin conditions can be irritating for both men and women. However, benign prostatic hyperplasia can be a major problem for men, and it can also be irritating for those who have a husband, father, brother, or son who may be battling this condition. It is usually age related, beginning in middle age. Enlargement of the prostate can block the flow of urine out of the bladder, and the symptoms, which can range from having to urinate more often to having difficulty starting

to urinate, can be haunting for men. But it can be treated, and sometimes with superfoods.

What Superfoods Rx to Use: Eat ¼ cup of pumpkin seeds each day.
These little seeds can be eaten plain, in cereal, on top of salads, or
even in muffins and smoothies.

Why You'll Feel Supercharged: Cucurbitacins are compounds in
pumpkin seeds that may stop testosterone from morphing into a stronger
form of the hormone, which may keep the hormone from producing
enlargement of the prostate. Pumpkin seeds contain the mineral zinc.
Consuming these seeds may lessen the size of the prostate and relieve
bladder symptoms of benign prostate hyperplasia.[4]

38. PSORIASIS (CHASE AWAY ITCHINESS)

Like poison ivy and poison oak, another skin challenge is psoriasis,
which is a chronic condition in which skin cells turn into red, itchy
patches. These trouble spots most often show up on your hands, elbows, and legs. Living in the mountains, there is not a lot of humidity.
Dry hair and dry skin have paid me a visit, especially in the wintertime. One time, I went to the dermatologist, thinking I had a bout of
psoriasis. I did not; it was simply dry skin. If you have a mild case (not
severe) of either condition, superfoods can come to the rescue.

What Superfoods Rx to Use: Try a store-bought body soap or lotion
with both oats and yogurt.

Why You'll Feel Supercharged: Both oats and yogurt found in lotions
and body soaps contain anti-inflammatory compounds that can soothe
the itch and lessen the burn of skin conditions such as dry skin, poison
oak and poison ivy, and even a sunburn. Researchers believe the antioxidant, anti-inflammatory compounds in oats, called avenanthra-
mides, may soothe itching and irritated skin. You may experience
smoother and clearer skin, especially if it's a mild flare-up and is
treated regularly with this easy superfood home remedy.

39. SEASONAL AFFECTIVE DISORDER (LIGHTEN IT UP)

Welcome to the change of seasons. The term *seasonal affective disorder* describes how people's moods are adversely affected by the dark skies and lack of sunlight during the daytime in the fall and winter months. The term was coined by Dr. Norman Rosenthal, who knows firsthand about the scourge of cold, dark fall and winter days, and he has found ways to help people cope better during these times of year. Years ago, a friend of mine and I both battled the wintertime blues. We became "bad" carb buddies and would go on donut runs at night to deal with the low mood. However, once I moved to the cold wintertime setting in the Sierras, I followed the good doctor's advice.

Some helpful, practical tips I turn to are: turning up the thermostat, making a fire, letting more light in by opening the blinds in the daytime, turning on more lights at night, layering furniture with fluffy throws, and adding plants. But there is more you can do.

What Superfoods Rx to Use: Eat a hot, baked potato, sweet or russet variety, once a day for lunch or dinner.

Why You'll Feel Supercharged: Research done at the Massachusetts Institute of Technology in Cambridge shows that starchy carbohydrates found in potatoes can rev up the feel-good serotonin chemical, reducing hunger pangs and calming you to stave off stress eating and boost your mood. Not only does this home cure work at home, but the funny thing is, it also does its job anywhere. These days I adore overcast days and rainstorms on the West Coast, in the Pacific Northwest, and even when I traveled to Quebec. If you combine the practical tips with superfoods, it may surprise you and boost your mood, too! Also, instead of munching on empty-calorie junk food, turn to superfoods (such as fruits and vegetables) for energy and calmness.

Getting a Daily Dose of Sunshine Superfoods

Vitamin D is important for good health. If you live in a region that gets less sun rather than more, or if you're not outdoors a lot, growing older, or a vegetarian, you may be lacking in the sunshine vitamin D. So, how do you get it without taking a vitamin supplement? Sunshine superfoods can help!

A serving of fortified whole-grain cereal contains 35 percent of your daily requirement of vitamin D. Another 15 percent of recommended vitamin D is in organic milk and 25 percent in a serving of orange juice, which you can add to a smoothie. Getting an adequate amount of vitamin D each day (it varies depending on your age) helps enhance the immune system, bones, mood disorders, and overall good health and well-being.

40. SINUSITIS (CLEAR THE PASSAGES)

For decades, seasonal affective disorder has paid me visits, but I've learned to deal, whereas sinus woes still are a challenge. One winter on a Friday evening, I was battling postnasal drip. It was too late to go to the doctor and not bad enough to sit in the ER waiting room. So, I took a fourth antihistamine. Because I'm small, within less than an hour I suffered from severe cramping and multiple bathroom visits. Hours later, a call to the paramedics was made, and at midnight there was a knock at the front door.

I crawled out of bed, through the hallway, and into the living room to open the door. After telling the crew of five that it was the pills causing my physical woes, which were worse than the postnasal drip, they believed me, sort of. I didn't go to the hospital. The next day I vowed never to take the over-the-counter medication again. Instead, I turned to the superfoods cure.

What Superfoods Rx to Use: Homemade salsa made with chili peppers, fresh tomatoes, onions, and garlic—and water, water, water.

Why You'll Feel Supercharged: The hot peppers, onions, and garlic can help break up the mucous (the stuff in your throat) that causes congestion, open the airways, and allow you to breathe easier. Tomatoes are rich in antioxidants to help lower the risk of getting a sinus infection. The combination of the superfoods in salsa is a surefire (pun intended) remedy to keep your throat clear, headache away, and the paramedics at bay. Not to forget that drinking plenty of water (hot tea can be included) will help break up the postnasal drip in your throat and clear your sinuses.

41. SORE THROAT (LOSE THE PAIN)

Dealing with a bout of sinus problems is a challenge, but a sore throat is nothing to ignore, either. Often throat irritation comes on if you're talking too much, but the telltale sore throat before a cold is one you usually tend to ASAP. Yes, superfoods can be helpful and may lessen the pain and severity of it.

What Superfoods Rx to Use: Use fresh water and make a cup of hot tea and squeeze fresh lemon in it. Repeat as needed.

Why You'll Feel Supercharged: Throat lozenges coat your throat, but so does tea and lemon. What's more, thanks to the antibacterial properties of lemon, which is rich in the antioxidant vitamin C, it can actually heal a sore throat. Also, folk remedy proponents will tell you that drinking a glass of warm lemon water daily may lower the risk of developing a sore throat.

42. STRESS (TAME THE NERVES)

Nobody likes to feel stressed out, which can be linked to work, family, finances, or even illness in the family or yourself. There are anti-stress remedies, and one includes stress-busting foods. Nutritionists will tell you crunchy, nutrient-dense foods can help soothe frazzled nerves and are good for your health, too.

What Superfoods Rx to Use: Eat one apple every day.

Why You'll Feel Supercharged: The crunchy apple is nature's stress reducer and can instantly make you feel calmer. Also, the nutrients, including dietary fiber, will help keep you satisfied so you won't be tempted to overindulge in processed, sugary foods. Plus, apples can aid in keeping you regular, which may be a challenge during stressful times.

43. STYES (PAMPER THE HURT)

A reddish bump on your eyelid known as a stye (or pink eye) can be pesky, causing stress as well as hurt. Years ago, I did have one, but by the time I made a doctor's appointment, it had gone away by itself, as they sometimes can do. But if a minor stye pays you a visit, the superfood potato may be just the healing medicine needed to heal it.

What Superfoods Rx to Use: Wash and peel a warm russet potato. Cut a thin slice of the white part and wrap it in cheesecloth. Place it on the stye for fifteen minutes. Repeat three to four times daily.

Why You'll Feel Supercharged: Compounds in a potato can help reduce redness and inflammation. Plant-based foods like potatoes, called tubers, contain astringent, antibacterial, and anti-inflammatory properties that can lessen skin irritation, swelling, and redness. Also, the warm compress may help to soften and drain the inflamed tissue in the stye. If it works, you'll be pleased that you didn't have to go to the doctor or resort to taking some type of medication. Natural cures can do the job, and they're worth a try.

44. ACTINIC KERATOSES (COVER THAT SKIN)

Styes are not fun, whereas actinic keratoses, or AKs, can be dangerous if not treated. AKs are small, crusty, hard bumps on your skin, usually in spots that get a lot of sun. If not treated, they can become cancerous. One cold winter day, I was en route for a checkup with my general practitioner. In the office I asked, "What's this?" I pointed to the small red spot on my left cheek. Without hesitation he answered, "An AK." I was told it could be zapped with liquid nitrogen by him or the dermatologist. I did have the quick procedure done, and the spot has remained spotless.

What Superfoods Rx to Use: Eat one serving of niacin-rich poultry three times per week. Pair it with a fortified whole-grain cereal every day. (The recommended dietary allowance is 20 milligrams.)

Why You'll Feel Supercharged: I was told by the dermatologist's assistant that getting niacin (vitamin B₃) may be helpful in keeping AKs at bay. Past research has shown that people who lack vitamin B_3 (again, vegetarians may find it challenging to get an adequate amount) may be more prone to skin cancer, whereas getting the adequate amount (not more) can be helpful in keeping your skin cancer-free.

45. TENDONITIS (TAKE IT SLOW)

We need to keep an eye on our skin, but we also need to keep an eye out for problems with our arms and legs. One winter day, I vacuumed the cabin using a new, cumbersome vacuum cleaner. After, I headed to the swimming pool, where I swam laps, and then I walked my Australian shepherd (half my size). Later in the day, my right forearm (the one I favor for work and play) started to throb. Ah, tendonitis! Translation: This is when tendons, the bands of tissue that are connected to muscles and bones, become tender due to repetitive injury and overuse. Guilty as charged and in pain.

What Superfoods Rx to Use: Bring out the ice pack (yes, superfood water again!), and place it on the painful area for about 15 minutes three to four times per day.

Why You'll Feel Supercharged: Enduring a forearm that has a dull ache and burning sensation is not fun. Using cold ice helps to numb the pain as well as lessen tissue inflammation and heal the injury. Likely, using the arm more rather than less (not just overdoing it all at once) and warming up before exercise is wise in a perfect world. In an imperfect and hectic world, sometimes we have to treat our wounds and learn the hard way. Thank goodness for the superfood water and its superpowers.

46. TOOTHACHE (NUMB THE THROBBING)

When your limbs ache, it's a challenge, but an achy tooth? Sometimes, it may not even be the tooth that is the culprit and cause of the throbbing. Often, it may be a minor gum issue in the bothersome spot. If you find this is the case and it's on a weekend, after dental office hours, or a holiday, you're not out of luck. There is a superfood solution.

What Superfoods Rx to Use: Try rinsing the affected area with a mixture of warm salt water. Also, an ice cube can help.

Why You'll Feel Supercharged: Water in a mixture or frozen is a natural fix that can work wonders. Sometimes, if you eat something hard like a chip or cookie, it can affect your gum temporarily. Using anti-inflammatory salt water and/or numbing it with an ice cube will provide instant relief and even heal the red or swollen gum tissue. It's natural and you may not need prescription antibiotics or those over-the-counter topical tooth remedies that do have potential side effects. Try the superfoods cure first.

47. UNIVERSAL EMERGENCY (STOCK UP SELF-RELIANCE)

A throbbing gum can seem like a natural disaster, but so can a cold, sore throat, stomachache, or even frazzled nerves. When the lights go out or worse, don't forget to have a superfoods stash on hand. Bottled, canned, and dried foods work best.

What Superfoods Rx to Use: Water, dried fruits, nuts, nut butters, pasta, seeds, whole-grain crackers and cereals, canned fish, and fruit juices are all good superfoods to store. Use as needed.

Why You'll Feel Supercharged: Eating and drinking fresh food and water is best, but during times of need, nutrient-dense superfoods will suffice. Not only can they taste good, they'll also provide nourishment with essential vitamins and minerals and help keep you hydrated. Often, people will stock up on emergency foods that they do not like and thus will not be enjoyed or eaten in time of need.

48. URINARY TRACT INFECTION (PREVENT A FLARE-UP)

My grandmother, at age seventy-five, ended up in the hospital with a serious urinary tract infection (UTI). She blamed it on chemicals in bubble bath and made me vow I'd never use it. But I'm sensing she wasn't drinking enough water on a daily basis (not uncommon for elderly people, who can end up dehydrated), nor was the anti-UTI superfood cranberry juice part of her diet regime.

What Superfoods Rx to Use: Drink one 8-ounce glass of cranberry juice daily. Also, drink seven to eight 8-ounce glasses of water daily.

Why You'll Feel Supercharged: Past medical research has proven that both cranberry juice and water can help keep bacteria at bay, so a UTI is less likely to happen. Past research also shows that cranberries contain anti-inflammatory and antibacterial components such as phytonutrients (anthocyanins, catachins, lutein, and quercetin). If you're a woman who is prone to getting UTIs, look at what may be the cause, including hormonal changes with age that result in vaginal atrophy, making skin tissue more vulnerable to bacteria. It's key to know that the natural cranberry cure is most useful as a preventative measure instead of a treatment or remedy. Also note, cranberry juice is not recommended for women and men who suffer from interstitial cystitis flare-ups (inflammation of the bladder), as it can actually be a trigger food.

49. WARTS (SHRINK THE BUMP)

No, a wart on your hand or foot is not a disaster, but it can seem like one if a big event is coming up for you and you have to reveal skin. Plantar warts can end up on the soles of your feet (walking barefoot around a swimming pool or locker room is one way to get the virus that causes them), whereas warts also can pop up on your fingers or toes, usually. You can go to the dermatologist and have a wart sprayed with liquid nitrogen, known as cryotherapy to remove it (sometimes it has to be done again later), or you can try to take the natural route for good results, too.

What Superfoods Rx to Use: Place a slice of raw russet potato on the wart and cover it with a Band-Aid or duct tape. You can follow up with a bit of apple cider vinegar to expedite the effect of the superfoods remedy.

Why You'll Feel Supercharged: Potatoes—the white part and skins— can and do work, according to people who love and use folk remedies for pesky skin woes like warts. Anecdotal evidence shows this home cure may work to get rid of the wart because covering it with the potato can keep air from getting to it. One summer, I tried covering a plantar wart on my foot, but instead of a potato I used apple cider vinegar. The superfood remedy did its job.

50. WOUNDS (HEAL THE SORE)

Warts are unwelcome visitors, but wounds are worse because they can be prone to infection. One night, while sleeping, I was quickly awakened by my dog, who was spooked by a sound outside. Two raccoons sitting on the fence were staring at us through the bedroom window. My protective canine's attentive behavior of barking frightened the cat, who fled and scratched my right wrist and arm. Still sleepy, I wasn't sure what home cure to turn to, and I dealt with the damage with superfoods in the morning.

What Superfoods Rx to Use: Wash a scratch with soap and water to keep it clean. Put a paste of oats, honey, and water on top of it a few times per day. Use oatmeal-based soap to heal the scab.

Why You'll Feel Supercharged: Oatmeal is soothing, especially in a body lotion or body wash, and you can get brands that are designed for sensitive skin. No irritation, and oatmeal will help heal and smooth out the scratch, helping speed up the healing process, and it's gentle.

SUPER-IOR HEALING SUPERFOODS FOR THOUGHT

Ailment	Superfood	What It May Do
√ Actinic keratosis	Poultry, whole-grain cereal	Protects against sun damage
√ Allergies	Apples, berries, nuts	Eases symptoms from allergens
√ Anemia	Shellfish	Aids in energy, boosts red blood cells
√ Anxiety	Cranberries and yogurt	Reduces stress, calms nervous system

Ailment	Superfood	What It May Do
√ Asthma	Water, tomatoes	Opens airways, detoxifies body
√ Autoimmune disorders	Sea vegetables	Bolsters immune system
√ Blues	Chocolate, nuts, and seeds	May boost spirit
√ Brain fog	Walnuts	Improves alertness
√ Canker sores	Water, Greek yogurt	Soothes the pain, heals the skin
√ Clogged	Grape or pomegranate juice	Maintains healthy blood flow in arteries
√ Cold and flu	Chicken vegetable soup	May speed recovery, prevent illness
√ Constipation	Lemon water	Helps regularity
√ Cough	Chamomile tea, lemon, and honey	Controls coughing
√ Dehydration	Water	Aids hydration
√ Dental cavities	Yogurt and/or cheese	Helps coat teeth
√ Depression	Fruit and tea	Boosts mood
√ Diarrhea	Blueberries and yogurt	Aids digestive problems
√ Dizziness	Water	Helps steady you
√ Fibromyalgia	Cranberries	Helps reduce pain
√ Food poisoning	Water and apple cider vinegar	May prevent illness

Ailment	Superfood	What It May Do
√ Gingivitis	Yogurt	Helps reduce inflammation
√ Headache	Chicken or turkey	Provides relief and prevents pain
√ Heartburn	Yogurt	Aids in discomfort
√ Herpes	Seaweed	Lessens a flare-up
√ High blood pressure	Berries and melons	Helps to keep heart healthy
√ Infections	Maple syrup	Acts as an immunity booster
√ Insomnia	Yogurt and honey	Enhances tranquility
√ Jet lag	Lemon water, nuts	Provides energy
√ Kidney stones	Water	May help prevent blockage
√ Lackluster libido	Apples and water	Aids in boosting sex drive
√ Morning sickness	Yogurt	Lessens queasy feeling
√ Muscle pain	Ice, cherry juice	Soothes the ache
√ Panic attack	Water (tea)	Stops the anxiety
√ Plaque, tartar	Cheese	Protects against buildup
√ Poison oak/ivy	Oats	Relieves burning/itching
√ Prostate problems	Pumpkin seeds	May stave off prostate enlargement
√ Psoriasis	Oats and yogurt	Soothes redness, itching

Ailment	Superfood	What It May Do
√ Prostate problems	Pumpkin seeds	May stave off prostate enlargement
√ Psoriasis	Oats and yogurt	Soothes redness, itching
√ Seasonal affective disorder	Potatoes	Fights stress and sadness
√ Sinusitis	Hot tomato salsa	Clears airways and lessens congestion
√ Sore throat	Lemon water	Relieves soreness
√ Stress	Apple	May calm frazzled nerves
√ Stye	Potato	Relieves inflammation, soreness
√ Tendonitis	Ice	Relieves pain temporarily
√ Toothache	Water (salt)	Fights the infection
√ Universal emergency	Fruit, nuts, nut butters, seeds, whole-grain crackers, water	Provides energy, well-being, and survival
√ Urinary tract infection	Cranberry juice, water	Acts as a preventative medicine
√ Warts	Potato	Dries up warts
√ Wounds	Oats, honey, yogurt	Fights infection, soothes pain

PART 5

SUPERFOOD MANIA

Beautifying Superfoods

Though we travel the world to find the beautiful,
we must carry it with us, or we find it not.
—RALPH WALDO EMERSON, *Essays,* "Art"

During a calming trip to Victoria, British Columbia, looking for a Mediterranean climate and place to stay lean while I tried to get the peace I had longed for, a surprise caught me off guard. I noticed the town closed down early, yet it was still light out at 10:00 P.M., leaving me with *Insomnia*-like images of Al Pacino's film character trying to adapt to long hours of daylight in Alaska during the summer months. Worse, the hotel did not offer pay-per-view movies, nor did I bring a book. To make the best of the quietude, I decided it was a sign for some beauty-pampering me time.

I took strawberries (offered in the concierge's dinner/appetizers room) and mashed them up in a cup. I put up my hair and massaged the red, juicy goo on my face, which was a bit sun-kissed from the day on the boat and wharf. Fifteen minutes later, I rinsed the superfruit mask off. It was amazing to see my skin look more vibrant and feel smoother despite the day of wind and sun at the ocean. True, there wasn't anyone except me to admire the beautifying moment of beauty, but it was a sweet strawberry thing to remember during the sounds of silence in Victoria.

HEAD-TO-TOE BEAUTY REMEDIES

At home or on vacation, you can use an array of superfoods to beauty up from head to toe. Not only are some nutrient-dense foods inexpensive, they're readily available in your kitchen.

HAIR

Lemons, yes, fresh lemon juice, can be used to cope with dry hair or dandruff flakes. Also, if you want to lighten your blonde or light-brown locks, lemon can provide highlights. Put lemon juice on your hair and sit in the sunshine for about 30 minutes. (Wear sunscreen on your body and face.) Rinse. Dry. Yes, I can personally attest that this tip does brighten and lighten brown hair.

Turkey is another superfood to help your crowning glory. No, it's not to be used topically, but while using home remedies, it could help to eat a turkey salad or sandwich on whole-grain bread. Since your hair is 97 percent protein and 3 percent water, hair nutrition experts agree that a diet rich in protein is key to a thick, shiny mane. Protein-rich turkey builds amino acids that strengthen hair.

FACE

Dull skin: An egg white, whisked, then rubbed on your face until it dries can work wonders. Wash it off, pat dry. Your face will feel smooth and vibrant.

Smooth It: Combine 1 tablespoon milk, 1 tablespoon maple syrup, and 2 tablespoons oatmeal, ground finely. Spread on face and neck. Rinse after 15 minutes, pat dry. Apply moisturizer.

Pore Reducer: You can decrease unsightly pores with tomatoes! Add 2 tablespoons tomato juice to 1 tablespoon water. Spread on your face. Rinse off after 5 minutes, pat dry. The vitamin C and other antioxidants will give your face a rosy red glow.

EYES

Dark circles: If you're tired of looking at the raccoon-like rings under your eyes, you're probably interested in finding a solution that works. Sometimes darkened skin in this tender spot on your face can be due to a lack of shut-eye, a poor diet, or your mother. If genes are not to blame and it's temporary (from stress, not getting a good night's sleep, or a vacation), superfoods may help lighten the darkness. Try placing slices of raw potato under your eyes. Repeat morning and night. It is believed the raw potato cure can work because of its potassium content, which can help lighten the darker skin.

ELBOWS

Lemons may be the number-one beautifying superfruit because of their multiple uses and benefits. If you've noticed that your elbows feel rough and not soft, lemons may be the answer. Try this home remedy, shared by nutritionist Robin Foroutan, R.D., spokesperson for the Academy of Nutrition and Dietetics: After you've sliced a lemon in half, squeeze the juice out. Then place your elbows into each half lemon for about 10 to 15 minutes. The acids in the lemon will loosen the dry skin. Add sugar to the lemon halves because it works like a scrub. You can also use a loofah or washcloth to exfoliate your elbows.

FEET

Eggs and lemon can be nourishing, not only to the face but also to your feet! Combine 1 egg yolk with 2 tablespoons sesame oil and 2 tablespoons olive oil. Add 1 tablespoon fresh lemon juice and 1 tablespoon apple cider vinegar. Gently rub the mixture on your entire foot. Leave on for 20 minutes, then rinse with cool water. Pat dry and apply an oats-and-yogurt moisturizer. (A ready-made product can contain colloidal oatmeal to help smooth the skin and replenish moisture by acting as a skin protectant.)

SUPERFOODS SPA BEAUTY TREATMENTS MENU

Hotel spa menus include superfoods to drink and eat, and for spa treatments, too. A breakfast menu at the Marriott or Hyatt chains often offers a variety of fresh juices, including cranberry, orange, and tomato, which are included in the top 20 superfoods, as are breakfast foods such as berries, whole-grain breads and cereal, eggs, and melons.

Hotel spas in the United States and other countries are privy to superfood beauty treatments. (I do favor the Marriott and Hyatt hotels, but have stayed at pet-friendly chain motels and quaint B-and-Bs.) Some of these special pampering services include berry manicures and seaweed wraps. Since spas in your hometown or elsewhere can merge or change names, I'm providing some spa treatments you may find available no matter wherever you go.

- ✓ **The Body Scrub:** A spa in Vermont offers a maple sugar body scrub. The entire body is polished with real maple sugar made from Vermont maple trees, which may give patrons the ultimate hydrating experience.
- ✓ **The Body Scrub:** In Northern California, you can get a lemon scrub. Using juice from a local Meyer lemon, lemon olive oil, and sea salt, it may be the ultimate natural body exfoliating scrub.
- ✓ **The Body Wrap:** In exotic Jamaica, a spa offers a Broccoli and Aloe Vera Wrap for its antiaging and hydrating healing powers. It is poured and brushed onto the skin. After, a dip in an infinity swimming pool, with its healing water, tops off the superfood spa experience.
- ✓ **The Body Wrap:** A spa in Australia provides a Honey and Almond Wrap. It is a body exfoliation using a blend of ground almonds, honey, and warm water.
- ✓ **The Body Wrap:** In the Pacific Northwest, a Seaweed Nourishing Wrap is offered to help in recharging energy levels using the vitamins and minerals in seaweed to aid in detoxification.
- ✓ **The Body Beverages:**—In the Gulf States, a spa serves up healthful smoothies and juices, including antioxidant-rich ones with apples.

A Day in a Life with a Superfoods Devotee

Whether you live in the mountains, city, suburbs, or a rural town, superfoods can be infused into ready-made body lotions, facials, and shampoos. Also, you can prepare your own superfoods, from juices to smoothies and salads to soup—all whisking you far away to bliss without traveling outside of your home.

Take a peek at a day in my life after spending time in Superfoods-land. Always a superfoods lover, I have discovered a lot of how superfoods can be added to my own beauty regime, and you may, too!

8:00 A.M.: Drink a glass of water with fresh lemon juice. Brew a cup of coffee. Instead of fortified orange juice, squeeze oranges and grapefruits for juice. Make a bowl of oatmeal topped with fresh berries and nuts.

8:30 A.M.: Shower with an oats-and-yogurt–based body lotion from head to toe. Use an oatmeal-based lotion after drying off.

9:00 A.M.: Second feeding for the dog. (He likes to graze on good grub, like mom.) Use the all-natural superfood dog food.

11:00 A.M.: Go to the resort pool. Swim laps; use the hot tub. Drink the citrus-infused water. Sip bottled water on the way home to rehydrate.

Noon: Warm up homemade vegetable and whole-grain noodle soup. Pair with artisanal whole-grain bread. Toss together a salad mix of kale and spinach with tomatoes, olive oil, and red wine vinegar.

1:00 P.M.: Feed the dog again; later take him for a walk and our exercise. More water for both of us upon arrival home.

2:00 P.M.: Work at home. Drink herbal tea. Eat an apple for a snack.

5:00 P.M.: Eat baked chicken with a baked potato and cruciferous vegetables on top.

6:00 P.M.: Drink a cup of black or white tea and continue working. Make a fire. Apply oats-based lotion on hands to keep them smooth due to the wood fire and dry air, lack of humidity.

8:00 P.M.: Call it a night and take time to relax. Brush dog. Brush dog's and cat's teeth as well as my own. Floss. Eat a handful of grapes or an orange. Drink a cup of chamomile tea.

10:00 P.M.: Climb into bed and watch TV. Turn off all the lights by midnight to get seven hours of rejuvenating sleep.

I may have inspired you to incorporate superfoods into your own day-to-day beautifying lifestyle. Once you go clean, eat real food, and use natural products infused with superfoods, it will be a challenge to turn back. It's time to take a quality-time break with a smoothie!

Super Beautifying Crowning-Glory Cantaloupe Smoothie

❖ ❖ ❖

This beautiful hair-inspired recipe was created for a variety of reasons. Years ago, I wrote an article on hair and how to put your diet to work to help enhance your locks. I went to hair experts and nutritionists and discovered a lot about what nutrients are essential for shiny and soft hair. For starters, vitamin A (cantaloupe) is necessary for oil production in the scalp, vitamin C (pineapple) aids in iron absorption, which prevents iron deficiency that would lead to hair loss, and vitamin E (wheat germ) retards aging of hair cells.

Protein plays a big role in beautiful, strong hair. Essential fatty acids (almonds, shellfish) keep hair nourished and soft. Also, protein (cheese, yogurt) builds amino acids that strengthen hair.

Not to forget that calcium (cheese and yogurt) makes hair healthier and stronger. And zinc, another hair-helping mineral (shellfish), aids in formation of skin and hair proteins.

And these essential nutrients are in my favorite superfoods. Go ahead—whip up a smoothie to help keep your hair healthy. Bottoms up.

½ cup organic half-and-half

¼ cup organic low-fat almond milk

½ cup premium vanilla gelato

½ cup cantaloupe, cubed

½ cup fresh pineapple juice

½ cup banana slices

1 tablespoon nut butter (your choice)

1 tablespoon wheat germ

2 tablespoons protein powder

4–5 ice cubes

1 teaspoon raw honey or maple syrup

Almonds, sliced, for topping

Fresh mint leaves for garnish

Put all ingredients including half-and-half, milk, gelato, fruit, nut butter, wheat germ, protein powder, ice, and syrup in a blender. If it has a "smoothie" button on it, all the better. Blend until thick but not too thin. Pour into glasses. Top with nuts and mint, and use a straw and spoon. You can put the smoothies in the freezer for 15–20 minutes to make them colder.

Makes 2 servings.

You've got the idea about how superfoods can be a beautifying experience, but why stop there? I adore having my home earthy and cozy. Enter superfoods. Real foods from nature can help you to enhance a happy, healthy, and balanced household. Discover in the next chapter exactly how superfoods can also beautify your environment, room by room, both indoors and outdoors.

SUPER-IOR HEALING SUPERFOODS FOR THOUGHT

✓ Superfoods can help exfoliate and soften your skin and make your skin and hair healthier, whether you do it yourself or get "spa'd" at a day spa or resort spa.

✓ Beauty treatments using superfoods (including berries, lemon, seaweed, and water) vary and are used in a variety of facial masks, body wraps, manicures, pedicures, and baths, which are offered at spas in the United States and around the world.

✓ Superfoods often include antibacterial and anti-inflammatory compounds that can be used on your body from head to toe for soothing and smoothing beautifying benefits, and they have been appreciated since the beginning of time.

✓ Eating clean, real superfoods throughout the day can help you feel and look your best.

Superfoods for a Healthy Household

*The best time for planning a book is while you're
doing the dishes.*

—AGATHA CHRISTIE

Before my last Canada R-and-R getaway, the upset of leaving my cozy
cabin and canine, a devoted Australian shepherd, Skyler, was the
biggest feat for me. I felt the void in my household. Despite leaving
him to caring attendants, complete with bag of superfood dog chow,
toys, brushes, and oatmeal-based shampoo, I was coping with separa-
tion anxiety. I checked with the kennel with a follow-up call in the afternoon to see how he was doing; we both were down. But this time
around, my cat, Zen, licked the salty tears on my cheeks, and once I
was in a Zen-like state, it gave me time to clean the cabin and bake
superfoods to freeze so homemade fresh fruit and nut muffins and
scones would greet me upon my return.

I depleted the refrigerator of fruits and vegetables and cleaned the bathroom (kitty litter box, too). Turning to lemon, water, and white vinegar—no toxic fumes from commercial cleaners was the answer to super cleaning. After the rooms were in order, it was time to get my bags and paperwork ready to go. And to this day, I recall the fresh scent of lemon and lavender lingering in the air. It was heaven, but being "dogless," there was a void, the worst part of traveling.

SUPERFOODS FOR YOUR HOME—ROOM BY ROOM

INSIDE THE LIVING ROOM

Conceal flaws naturally. If you have a favorite sofa or love seat made with wood, it's frustrating when surface scratches taint your beloved piece of furniture due to wear and tear. I tried rubbing a shelled walnut on the wood to mask the unsightly imperfections. It seemed to conceal to a scratch or two, but it wasn't perfect. I decided to eat the nuts and live with the character flaws.

DINING ROOM

Add bowls of fresh fruit. Superfruits, such as red apples and green apples, add life to the dining room when it's being used for entertainment. In the film *The Break-Up*, Jennifer Aniston's character, Brooke Meyers, got flustered when her partner didn't bring enough lemons home from the store to be used for an elegant centerpiece on the table.

EARTHY KITCHEN

Display nature's cleaners. Use lemon and water. In a spray water bottle, add the juice from one fresh lemon, 2 tablespoons white vinegar, and fill it up with tap water. This can be used to clean countertops, inside the microwave, and on top of the oven. It cuts through dirt and grease, leaving a nice fragrance.

Provide a water spritzer. A water bottle on the countertop is a great way to keep healthy plants green and thriving.

NATURAL BEDROOM

Provide a water pitcher. Add water in a container on top of a dresser or by the bed. Drinking water first thing in the morning is a healthful practice to get used to doing, plus the pitcher adds a fresh look and feel by adding nature's super superfood.

SCENTED BATHROOM

Use nature's soaps. In the shower or by the tub, add superfood beauty products for a down-to-earth healthy vibe. My shower includes a body wash infused with oatmeal. Bar soaps include extracts of oatmeal and citrus.

Scrub with green cleaners: To clean an enamel sink or toilet, try an all-natural homemade lemon scrub. Combine juice from one fresh lemon with ½ cup all-natural laundry soap.

HOME OFFICE

Add water. A drinking-water device is a good idea. It will add a superfood element and remind you to include water in your daily diet at work. Using water infused with fruit will make it more appealing to the eye and tastier to the palate.

Maintain a water decoration. Trickling water in a natural fountain is a way to keep nature inside and maintain a sense of calm for you and visitors. Dentist's and doctor's offices as well as health spas often contain flowing waterfall objects.

KEEP IT GREEN OUTDOORS

Wash the windows. Cleaning windows with an ammonia-based cleaner works, but the scent is less than desirable. Try making your own window cleaner: mix 1 cup water, ½ cup white vinegar, and 2 tablespoons lemon juice. It works, perhaps not as well as a streak-free commercial cleaner, but its fragrance makes up for a streak or two.

Compost for nature. Transform waste into a rich soil. It's an eco-friendly action. Recycle superfoods waste to keep outdoor plants and foliage healthy. Place eggshells (crushed), and seaweed (thin layers) onto soil for best results.

HOUSEHOLD CLEAN-UP WITH SUPERFOODS

Superfoods are super, but sometimes they end up in places that we don't want them to be or they can be used to get rid of other foods that need to go. Here, take a look.

Lemon for unwanted stains: Superfruit lemons boast antiseptic and antibacterial healing powers, especially when it comes to zapping stains. Both lemon juice and peels can act like bleach (but more gentle) and be used to get rid of food spots on carpets or clothing.

Potatoes for rust: No kidding. Basic russet potatoes are recommended to help get rid of rust. Peel a medium-sized potato and dip the white super vegetable into mild dish soap. Scrub the rusted area on outdoor furniture, wheelbarrows, or any metal objects. Repeat until the rust is gone. I did try this remedy on a black wrought-iron chair sitting on the deck.

Tomatoes for metals: And tomatoes are rust busters, too! Thanks to their acidity, they can help remove rust and tarnish from precious metals, silverware, and brass. Use tomato paste or juice. Rub it gently on the metal, leave on for several minutes, rinse off with water, dry, and buff. I tried this with a brass container. It did seem to get rid of the tarnish and made the piece shine.

Water for gum on furniture or carpets (or hair): It happens. If chewing gum gets stuck in any of these locations, H_2O comes to the rescue. Simply apply an ice cube (put it in a plastic bag) to the affected region. Freeze the gum. Repeat as needed.

Peanut butter for gum on pet or human hair: If water doesn't do the trick for hair, peanut butter (yes!) might work. Let a bit of the butter soak into the hair, remove it with a cloth, wash the hair, and rinse.

SUPERFOODS FENG SHUI

Using superfoods in feng shui is nothing new; in fact, the placement of healthy food goes back centuries, thanks to this Chinese art. There are many goals of using and arranging fruits, vegetables, and nuts in the house, which may bring you good health, harmony, and peace.

Citrus cleaners: Putting to work cleaning agents with citrus essential oil will provide a lingering, clean scent, but also it's eco-friendly and will give you better health and energy than using cleaning products with toxic ingredients.

Scents pot it up, naturally: A simmering potpourri can provide a wonderful aroma in your home. Try combining superfoods, including 3 cups water and 2 lemons with peels. Place them in a pot. Add spices, such as cinnamon and vanilla. Heat to a boil and then turn down the heat to a simmer for 20 minutes. Your kitchen will smell sublime any season of the year.

Seven lemons in a bowl: Like putting nine oranges in a bowl or basket, lemons are similar. Not only are they symbolic of good health, but of good energy, too. They last for quite a while (fresh is always best), look beautiful with their splash of yellow, and give a clean look and feel on a table or countertop.

Nine green apples in a basket: Apples, another superfruit, are relatively inexpensive, and placing green ones in a container provides many potential good-for-you images that may help you attain good health, prosperity, and peace.

Nuts with shells in a container: A mix of nuts, including Brazil nuts, peanuts, and walnuts, is attractive, with their different shapes and earthy colors. If you have kids or pets, please use a lid and put them up out of reach. Not only is this a reminder to use nuts in baking, cooking, and snacking, it's also a gift of nature that promises well-being and good fortune (especially the round-shaped nuts).

Trail mix in glass containers: When I used to clean homes to pay my way through graduate school, one woman (down-to-earth like me, but

I was penniless while she was wealthy) put together tall glass jars filled with homemade trail mix, including nuts, seeds, dried fruit, and carob chips. They are eye-friendly; however, only place them on countertops out of reach of young children and pets.

Water-fruit drinking container: At spas and dentist's offices, it's not uncommon to see a large container of water filled with slices of citrus fruit. I love doing this in the summer, but it can be used year-round to help you and yours to remember to stay hydrated.

A bonus superfoods tip: Put a framed picture of superfoods on your kitchen wall. This can be an array of nature's finest foods: fruits, vegetables, cheeses, breads, and wines—a splash of color reminding you of the healthful plant-based diet.

Healthy Kid Stuff

Kid-Friendly Superfood: Grilled Flatbread Pizza with Hidden Veggie Sauce

It's hard to get some kids to eat their veggies, but nearly all kids love pizza. The hidden vegetable tomato sauce in this recipe packs eggplant, carrots, celery, onion, garlic, and herbs into a rich pizza sauce that both kids and adults will eat up!

For the Hidden Veggie Sauce

½ cup extra-virgin olive oil

2 cups eggplant, peeled and diced small

1 cup onion, diced small

1 cup carrots, diced small

1 cup celery, diced small

2 or 3 garlic cloves, chopped

3 quarts canned crushed tomatoes (3 each, 28- or 32-ounce cans)

2 tablespoons fresh
  thyme, chopped
2 tablespoons fresh basil

1–2 dry bay leaves
Salt and pepper, to taste

For the grilled flatbread

Hidden Vegetable Tomato
  Sauce
Extra-virgin olive oil, as
  needed
Mozzarella, grated
Parmesan Reggiano,
  grated

Peasant bread (or any
  type artisanal crusty
  bread, whole-grain rec-
  ommended). [Use por-
  tion control for serving
  size of the flatbread.
  Portions can vary on
  age and size.]

In a large (5-quart or bigger) thick-bottomed pot, heat the olive oil over medium heat. Add the eggplant, onion, carrot, celery, and garlic and sauté gently (not browning vegetables or garlic) until the vegetables start to become tender. Add the tomatoes, herbs, and bay leaves. Simmer uncovered for about 1 hour, season to taste with salt and pepper. Puree until all vegetables are hidden in the tomato sauce. Chill and reserve to make quick pizzas.

To make the pizzas, preheat oven to 350 degrees F and preheat gas grill or grill pan to medium high. For each serving, cut 1 slice of peasant bread, sliced 1/4-inch to 3/8-inch thick. Brush bread generously with extra-virgin olive oil and season with salt and pepper. Spread the tomato sauce on the bread and grill it. Cover with grated mozzarella and sprinkle with grated Parmesan Reggiano. Bake in the oven until the cheese is melted, 10–15 minutes. Cut into wedges and serve.

Makes 3 quarts of sauce. Freeze in smaller portions for future use.

(Courtesy: North American Olive Oil Association, www.aboutoliveoil.com)

PETS AND SUPERFOODS

A super way to maintain your pet's youthful body and healthy state is by dishing up a high-quality or premium natural pet food. Holistic vets advise that chemicals found in typical supermarket commercial pet foods may up the odds of your pet developing cancer, cause liver or kidney damage, and even shorten a dog's or cat's life span.

The solution: Turn to an all-natural pet food complete with superfoods. That means a pet food diet that offers high quality, minimally processed ingredients without fillers, sugar, or chemical preservatives. Look for a food that lists at least two sources of protein and fat, such as chicken or fish, along with a good source of carbohydrates, such as whole rice or barley, and other essential nutrients.

Veterinarians have told me for years that a fresh, unprocessed diet based on natural, whole foods is healthful for dogs and cats. There is a downside of home cooking for your companion animals, however. The American Veterinary Medical Association warns that creating homemade pet food is not easy. Home-cooked pet foods are usually not created with the science commercial foods are, and the food can end up lacking key nutrients or not providing the right nutritional balance.

WHAT'S COOKING?

On the flip side, some people will turn to home cooking for their dogs and cats; there are countless recipes concocted by veterinarians. I've penned articles on this topic, and it can be done, but you risk leaving out key nutrients or using the wrong amounts, and it does take time.

I do dish up premium pet food to my dog and cat. I have read the food ingredients labels from the dog food my pooch has been eating since he was a pup. He is on a grain-free food processed with purified water. The chow includes smoked salmon, omega-3 fatty acids, potato fiber, blueberries and raspberries, and tomatoes. Sounds similar to my human list of the top 20 superfoods, doesn't it? My cat (half Siamese) had a bout of cystitis, which isn't uncommon in male cats. So, he has been on a special kidney-sensitive, low-ash, dry cat food diet, and fresh water has been available 24/7 for several years. He never had another episode, so while I'd prefer to dish up another superfood-type diet, since the one he is eating is doing its job, he will continue to eat the crunchy food.

In the twenty-first century, pets and humans both thrive on a nutrient-dense diet that includes superfoods. Check with your vet to see if your companion animal is on the best diet for its individual needs, and work together to achieve the best results. You can find an array of natural pet foods at pet shops, health food stores, and on the internet.

A house that is naturally healthy, complete with kids and pets, is full of life. Creating fun dishes for people of all ages makes it a super home. If you haven't tried making homemade frozen delights, take the ice cream maker challenge and enjoy making gelato with superfoods.

Super Cooling Berry Berry Gelato

❖ ❖ ❖

Add to the mix—kids and adults—and you've got more family fun, right? On a warm spring day or summer afternoon (or even on a chilly autumn or winter day), making gelato with an ice cream maker using superfoods is a super way to include kids in the art of cooking with healthful foods.

2 cups frozen fruit (a mix of berries: blackberries, blueberries, raspberries, strawberries)
2 tablespoons honey or maple syrup
1 cup organic low-fat milk
1 teaspoon pure vanilla extract
Sweet superfood toppings for garnish

In blender jar, mix ingredients, including fruit, honey, milk, and extract, together until the berry concoction becomes smooth. Pour into ice cream maker; follow manufacturer's directions. Serve in parfait glasses. I recommend providing different superfoods for toppings, including chocolate chips or whole berries. More choices offer more fun and adventure.

Makes 4 servings.

Nope, we're not done yet. It's time. It's time to get cooking! These superfoods that you're well versed in by now give even more. Sure, I teased with a recipe at the end of each chapter, but now here comes the real show, like a crescendo in a movie you've watched. Get cooking by mixing and matching all these superfoods. It's going to be like Fourth of July fireworks—but first, some details from storage to seasons and a sample diet plan you'll want to view before you hit the kitchen.

SUPER-IOR HEALING SUPERFOODS FOR THOUGHT

✓ If you have chemical sensitivities or care about using eco-friendly cleaning products inside and outside your home, superfoods are a healthful alternative.

✓ It's never too early to introduce your kids to eating superfoods. Start s-l-o-w-l-y. In other words, don't serve a superfood dark-green smoothie; whip one up kid-friendly with superfruits (add a bit of mixed lighter greens) and grow the young palate.

✓ Some—not all—superfoods can be super pet-friendly for better health and pet care.

✓ Superfoods can be used for arts and crafts in the household and are healthy in contrast with chemical-laden items.

✓ Cleaning the house with nature's finest, such as lemon and water, is much healthier for your house and you.

PART 6

SUPERFOOD RECIPES

The Joy of Cooking
with Superfoods

'Tis an ill cook that cannot lick his own fingers.
—WILLIAM SHAKESPEARE, *Twelfth Night*

A superfoods fest is part of my life, past and present, in and outside my home. Cooking with real, clean food is not only practical, it's also healing for the mind and body. One Thanksgiving at Lake Tahoe, I took an alternative route for a turkey dinner and all the trimmings. Instead of a family get-together or going out on the town, I cooked, but with a light touch.

Early in the morning, I woke up to no snow, no vacationing homeowners. I cuddled in bed with the Aussie and Siamese. In the afternoon, I watched movies and whipped together a dinner chock-full of superfoods, and while it was cooking, I made a fire for ambiance. No fuss, no mess. It was a simple but super plan. I didn't want to cook up a sixteen-pound turkey, so the menu consisted of two all-natural, organic game hens with a lemon herb glaze, chunky red mashed potatoes with chives, a kale-spinach and vinaigrette salad, whole-grain toasted French bread dipped in olive oil, and apple-cranberry crisp. The food boasted a Mediterranean flair with flavor and freshness. It was a joy to cook, a joy to eat. And this is how I put it together for Thanksgiving.

BEFORE YOU USE SUPERFOODS

Finding and purchasing superfoods is a process that you learn by trial and error. Once you discover the best source of superfoods, you'll want to store your favorite foods to ensure that you're preserving their quality. The adages "Waste not, want not" and "When in doubt, throw out" come into play. Here's proof.

When I was living in San Carlos, California, my girlfriend's teenage son visited me one day. He asked, "Got any eggs?" I paused and looked at the date of the carton in the fridge. "Expired," I answered and shrugged my shoulders. The young man took four eggs. He also inquired about potatoes. I pointed to a few white sprouts on the russet ones in a cupboard. He took the food and looked like he had found a treasure chest and took the superfoods back to his home. Less than a half hour later, I dropped in on him, standing over the stovetop in his mother's kitchen. I watched the resourceful young person morph into a chef. He diced his mom's onions, tomatoes, and cheese. Using spices, he added the eggs and potatoes (minus the sprouts). Within minutes, the story of the roasted potatoes and eggs from the children's book *The Secret Garden* by Frances Hodgson Burnett came to mind because "the eggs were previously a luxury and very hot potatoes with salt and fresh butter in them were fit for a woodland king." And that was the day I learned to use common sense before tossing food.

You don't have to toss some foods that are a bit past the expiration date, especially if you know the guidelines so you can still enjoy their healing powers.

No matter where you reside, whether it is the Golden State, like me, in New York City, in the middle states, or Alabama, or in Europe, you can hunt and find super superfoods—real, clean foods—to help you feel good.

When hunting and gathering superfoods at your supermarket, farmer's market, or from online sellers, please follow these tips:

- Find and check the "use by" date. Keep in mind, some foods, such as eggs or nuts, when stored properly can be used a bit longer than the expiration date.
- Check the source if you're purchasing cheese, fish, or poultry.
- Wash all fruit and vegetables (even prewashed packaged types) to lessen contact with pesticides.
- Choose organic produce, dairy, and poultry to get the healthiest foods without added ingredients.

Keeping your dried superfoods—including fruits, nuts, and seeds—in airtight containers inside a dark, cool pantry is the way you're told to do it. When I was gifted with berries, nuts, and seeds, it was tempting to try a variety. Once opened, however, I put the packages inside the refrigerator. Not only is this the way to do it for preservation, it also gave me peace of mind that the cat or dog wouldn't get into the superfoods. (Nuts, especially can be toxic to pets.)

You can be the final judge (there is no superfoods storage police force) on how to preserve your favorite superfoods. Also, you'll find that people will differ in their opinions on how to store certain foods. For instance, tomatoes can be put in the refrigerator vegetable bin, but some folks insist fresh tomatoes off the vine are best kept at room temperature. Whole-grain bread is superb when sitting on a cutting board waiting to be sliced; however, sometimes, I have stored breads—all types—in the fridge to keep them fresh longer. Rules are made to be broken, as my friend's son taught me with his superfoods breakfast that I almost passed up but got to enjoy, too.

Storing Superfoods at a Glance

Checking out the "best by" and expiration date of foods is a super guide, but there are exceptions. Storing superfoods in different ways (you're in charge) can help to maintain the integrity of the foods and their key nutrients and freshness for flavor and texture. Keeping superfoods in airtight containers and in the best places (which can be subjective) can help preserve their shelf life.

Superfood	Storage	Shelf Life
Dairy		
Eggs	Refrigerator	Up to 1 week after expiration date
Cheese	Refrigerator	Up to a few weeks after expiration date; toss if there is mold
Yogurt	Refrigerator	2 weeks–1 month
Fruits and vegetables		
	Refrigerator/room temperature	Varies depending on item
Avocados	Room temperature until soft	1–2 weeks
Fresh berries	Refrigerator	Up to 1 week
Leafy greens	Refrigerator	3 days–1 week
Lemons	Refrigerator	Up to 2 weeks
	Room temperature	7–10 days
Tomatoes	Cool, dry place	Up to 1 week
Grains (whole)		
All	Cool, dark place	1 week
Sweets		
Maple syrup	Cool, dark place	Up to 2 years
Nuts and seeds		
All	Cool, dark place; if opened, refrigerator	6 months–1 year
Water	Cool, dark place	Up to 1 year

SEASONAL SUPERFOODS AND FOUR SEASONS

WINTER

It's the Season: Growing up in the San Francisco Bay area, winter wasn't a chilly time; instead we were blessed with a Mediterranean-type climate. I recall playing hooky on school days as a kid and watching a TV show called *Candid Camera*, and seeing the East Coast's snow, which was foreign to me. Nowadays, after many winters living in the Sierra Nevada, I know what that white powder is, whether it be shoveling it, making a fire to keep toasty away from it, or baking comfort wintertime foods to forget it, including wholesome superfoods.

Healing Winter Recipes: Homemade bread, casseroles, and hearty soups and stews are part of a superfoods wintry diet. Including a variety of food groups—not just one or a few—can help you slim down, healthy up.

Winter Superfoods: Apples, berries (frozen, dried), cheese, maple syrup, pasta, pizza, whole-grain cereals.

SPRING

It's the Season: Living in the mountains brings four distinct seasons and four different ways of enjoying superfoods. Once the weather warms up, it's time to lighten up with superfoods and drop unwanted winter weight. A spike of energy happens and can be used along with superfoods in spring cleaning—indoors and outdoors—and in more play, from walking the dog to swimming in a warmer indoor pool.

Healing Spring Recipes: Meatless cooking is easier in the springtime because it's lighter on the body; it's a time to rejuvenate. Vegetarian casseroles, soups, and fruit smoothies to help cleanse and detox are all easy to prepare. Fresh fruits, instead of baking, used in vegetable and fruit salads work well to lighten up.

Spring Superfoods: Berries, eggs, leafy greens, lemons, Greek yogurt, pasta, seeds, shellfish, walnuts, and water.

SUMMER

It's the Season: During the hot summertime, easy no-cook meals and outdoor grilling are what people look forward to so they can enjoy more playtime. When the temperature soars, the last thing you want to do is bake or cook.

Healing Summer Recipes: Try cheese and fruit plates, cold fruit smoothies, Greek yogurt parfaits, cold cereals, vegetarian thin-crust pizza, poultry sandwiches, seafood salads, and iced tea.

Summer Superfoods: Berries, chicken, leafy greens, gelato, lemons, ice cream, pasta, tomatoes, water, and wine.

FALL

It's the Season: When the air gets colder and the leaves turn color, it's time to change some of your favorite superfoods. Apples, citrus, and first-time cooking feel right before the first fire is made and the thermostat is turned up. Warm food is beginning to replace the colder superfoods of summer.

Healing Fall Recipes: Apple pie, lemon-drizzled dishes, savory smoothies, hot oatmeal, and whole-grain pancakes with warm maple syrup all can help enhance the immune system. Also, pasta dishes, baked turkey and chicken, hot tea, fresh-squeezed juices, and hot apple cider can help you fill up, not out.

Fall Superfoods: Apples (harvest season, August–November), berries, crucifers, Greek yogurt, oats, turkey, seafood, sweet potatoes (harvest season, September–December), water, and wine.

THE HEALTH-BOOSTING SUPERFOODS FIVE-DAY MENU PLAN

This five-day "superfoods diet" is based on the nutrient-dense diet plans that a nutritionist and I created each week, years ago, when I was the diet and nutrition columnist for a national woman's magazine. However, back in the twentieth century when I cranked out these for our readers, it was common for me to squawk and squabble with the nutritionist when she would incorporate processed (tomato sauce and soup) and fat-free foods (cheese to yogurt). As a California nature girl, I wanted homemade sauces, soups, and real cheese and yogurt. Not to forget how I'd have a meltdown when meat was brought to the menu.

This diet plan is the way I ate decades ago and eat now, too. I'm dishing on organic, fresh, clean food from farm to table. I have enhanced the plan with heart-healthy superfoods found on the good-for-you food lists in the Mediterranean pyramid and foods chart. Diet plans, like this one, feature real food that can satisfy your palate and help you slim down and healthy up. This plan is timeless and full of deliciousness.

Recipes with an asterisk (*) can be found in previous chapters, especially at the end of each chapter, or in chapter 29, "Superfoods Menu." You can mix and match to suit your personal taste and custom-tailor it to the season.

Day 1: Fall

Breakfast:
　1 serving oatmeal with organic low-fat milk (fortified with calcium and vitamin D) and 2 tablespoons each nuts and dried or fresh berries
　1 serving fresh fruit juice
　Muffin
　1 boiled or scrambled egg

Lunch:
　1 serving Harvest Greens and Vinaigrette*
　1 Cherry-Almond Smoothie*

Snack:
　1 apple
　1 citrus-infused water or herbal tea

Dinner:
1 serving Lemon Chicken Breasts with Wild Rice and Crucifers*
1 serving greens
1 baked potato drizzled with olive oil and diced tomatoes
1 glass red wine or grape juice

Snack:
1 cube cheese
Fresh fruit (berries or apple)

Day 2: Winter

Breakfast:
1 serving whole-wheat pancakes drizzled with maple syrup
1 serving fresh-squeezed orange juice

Lunch:
1 serving Avocado, Strawberry, and Grilled Chicken Salad*

Snack:
1 serving Hidden Greens Smoothie*

Dinner:
1 serving Seafood Gumbo*
Artisanal whole-grain bread drizzled with olive oil

Snack:
1 serving Greek yogurt and nuts

Day 3: Spring

Breakfast:
1 serving Crunchy French Toast*
1 serving fresh berries

Lunch:
Quinoa Stuff(-ed) Pepper Bowl*

Snack:
  Cheese platter (cubes of cheese, crackers, grapes)

Dinner:
  Roasting Whole Cauliflower*
  1 serving vegetable salad

Snack:
  1 slice EVVO Lemon Cake*

Day 4: Summer

Breakfast:
  1 serving whole-grain fortified flakes with low-fat organic milk

Lunch:
  1 serving Dulse Miso Soup*
  1 serving watermelon-cheese salad: 1 cup watermelon, ¼ cup feta
    cheese, drizzled with olive oil and red wine vinegar, sprinkled
    with walnuts, garnished with fresh basil

Snack:
  1 serving Cinn-apple Smoothie*

Dinner:
  1 serving Flatbread Pizza*

Snack:
  1 serving ice cream or gelato and fresh berries

Day 5: All Seasons

Breakfast:
  1 serving Avocado Coconut Bowl with Pistachio-Coconut Granola*
  1 serving fresh juice (any variety)

Lunch:
 1 smoothie

Snack:
 1 serving Super-Duper Cheesy Potato Skins*

Dinner:
 Crispy Fish Filets in Oatmeal*
 1 serving spinach and kale salad with vinegar and olive oil

Snack:
 1 serving fresh fruit

Super Energizing Peanut Butter Fudge

I love peanut butter more than any nut butter. As the story goes, when I was a kid, after my mom returned from a trip to Europe, she was smitten with Mediterranean cuisine, from frog legs to snails. She used my siblings and me as lab rats and tried her dishes on our unsophisticated palates. More times than not, I, a picky eater, refused to oblige. Then she'd announce the punishment: "Peanut butter and jam sandwiches for dinner." I exhaled with relief. Nutty butter is like a reliable friend, it always comforts during the best and worst of times.

European-style butter
½ cup organic half-and-half
2 cups light brown sugar
1 cup all-natural peanut butter
1 teaspoon pure vanilla extract

3½ cups confectioners' sugar, sifted
½ cup each almonds and cashews chopped
¼ cup pumpkin, sesame, or sunflower seeds, shelled

In a saucepan melt butter on medium heat. Add brown sugar and milk. Stir in pan on stovetop for a couple of minutes until smooth. Remove from heat. Pour into a large bowl. Add peanut butter, vanilla extract, and sugar. Mix or beat mixture until creamy. Fold in nuts. In an 8-inch by 8-inch square pan, spoon in butter mixture and spread evenly. Top with seeds. Put in refrigerator for a few hours until firm. Take out and cut fudge into squares. Place in airtight container, store in refrigerator. Sugar is not a superfood! However, nuts, seeds, and nut butters are good for you. Enjoy in moderation.

Makes 16 pieces.

So, are you ready? Here comes the Superfoods Menu! I'm dishing up a variety of categories to show you how much fun you can have with superfoods. Imagine you're in the comfort of your home, but I'm giving you a hotel-type menu. Enjoy yourself and have fun creating superfoods meals all-year long. If you're short on time, whip up a smoothie!

SUPER-IOR HEALING SUPERFOODS FOR THOUGHT

✓ Eating superfoods without cooking, including salads, smoothies, and sandwiches, can be healthful, fun, and easy.
✓ Storing superfoods varies depending on whether you're eating fresh food, frozen, or dried. Expiration dates are super, but so is knowledge from the source where you get your superfoods.
✓ Seasons and superfoods are important. You can get some superfoods year round, but they can be pricey. It's best to buy and eat superfoods in season.

2 9

Superfoods Menu

The physician treats, but nature heals.
—HIPPOCRATES

When traveling throughout the United States and Canada, one of my favorite pastimes is to scan menus at hotels, in cafes, and even on trains. One trip to Quebec City in Via Rail Canada was a romantic Agatha Christie–type train ride through beautiful roadside views, where I once was too afraid to meet the destination because I didn't speak French. Before the trip, I chose business class, complete with a vegan dinner.

At dusk, when the conductor was serving up the meals, I was the only meatless passenger, he quickly pointed out. My superfoods meal, at first, seemed like a dream come true. It included a tomato-based vegetable and quinoa entree, honeydew melon and watermelon chunks, leafy greens with a balsamic vinaigrette, and a small multi-grain roll.

At first sight, the super array of superfoods looked appetizing. But, once I scrutinized the food choices, I was disappointed. The quinoa entrée (I still prefer brown rice) was sabotaged. Beans—not my favorite superfood, as noted earlier—were hiding beneath the vegetables and ancient grains. The salad was saturated in dressing, and the melon wasn't a warming food for the rare cold autumn. (A hot apple crisp would have been super.) I nibbled on the roll. When the conductor walked by me, he stopped. He stared at my food tray. "Madam? We prepared *your* vegan meal just for you." He shook his head, disappointed. This train-based dining scenario took me back to my childhood, when I refused to eat pea soup and Spam-like sandwiches at the babysitter's home. Blame it on the fuzzy beans and my superfood favorites. It didn't make the list.

Looking out the window at the amazing scenery, my mind wandered back home. I vowed that once I returned, I'd create a spin-off inspired by the French-style vegan dishes. Instead of quinoa, I'd use wild rice, fresh cruciferous vegetables, and tomatoes (not sauce)—beanless. The greens would be drizzled with extra-virgin olive oil and red wine vinegar. I'd serve hot oversized whole-grain rolls, and add a homemade apple-oats crumble with a scoop of vanilla gelato.

I reminisce now about the superfoods I did eat when in Quebec City. A cup of coffee (yes, this is a superfood, with its antioxidants) was a must-have before the horse and carriage ride I took to see the quaint town. Also, I stopped at a sandwich shop due to a bout of hunger and homesickness. I kept it simple and ordered a sandwich: one whole-grain roll, greens, tomatoes, Swiss cheese, olive oil and vinegar, and cut in half. No it wasn't fancy French food, but the simple superfoods made me feel good inside and outside as I appreciated the city that I once was too afraid to travel to when I had arrived in Montreal.

Decades later, I've discovered that when we travel, the foods we eat are part of the trip. Once back home, if we recreate what we ate, it's like revisiting the place, but in the comfort of our home, and controlling the superfoods in a dish is like enjoying the best of both worlds. Since I adore Canada, you'll find that many of the recipes that follow are inspired by the country in my heart.

THE HEALING POWERS SUPERIOR SUPERFOODS MENU

Cereal, Eggs, Muffins, Fresh Fruit

At home, fresh superfoods dished up for breakfast are ideal any season of the year. A bowl of hot steel-cut oatmeal topped with berries, fortified whole-grain cold cereal mixed with nuts and seeds, Florentine eggs, Greek yogurt and fresh melon chunks, quiche lorraine, or a berry-and-nut muffin are all worth writing home about, and you can create breakfasts in your own kitchen. Pair any of these superfoods with tea, coffee, and fresh juice, and you've got a super start for each and every day.

When time is not on your side, an Apple Oatmeal Muffin with Maple Syrup Frosting (made the day before) is perfect. An omelet infused with superfoods including real eggs, cheese, tomatoes, and vegetables is a comforting and filling breakfast at home, outdoors at a restaurant. or in a hotel room.

Don't ignore a basic bowl of plain Greek yogurt and seasonal fresh melon (drizzled with honey) to boost your energy, especially when paired with fresh-squeezed juice and a cup of coffee or tea. Yes, it's simple, but these superfoods are clean, real, and will nourish your body and spirit.

Apple Oatmeal Muffins with Maple Syrup Frosting
and Coffee
Avocado Coconut Bowl with Pistachio-Coconut Granola
and Fresh Juice
Blueberry Pancakes with Vermont Maple Syrup
and Herbal Tea
Citrus Muffins with a Twist and English Breakfast Tea
Greek Yogurt, Granola, and Seasonal Fresh Berries
and Black Tea

Apple Oatmeal Muffins with Maple Syrup Frosting and Coffee

Homemade muffins are easy to make and a ready-made breakfast food paired with fresh fruit. At Reno-Tahoe International Airport, I find myself more times than not taking an early morning flight. One time as I was waiting for a 6:00 A.M. flight, I ordered a coffee latte and banana nut muffin. The muffin was nondescript but do-able. I recall getting that familiar bout of homesickness, with thoughts like "I miss my dog," and then I went into future fantasy mode. I made a note to myself that once back home I'd bake a batch of apple muffins and include all the healthful ingredients. After I was introduced to amazing Vermont and Canadian maple syrup, I ended up more seasoned and added it to my California-style muffins.

FOR THE MUFFINS

2½ cups whole-wheat flour (O Organics)
¼ cup white granulated sugar or maple sugar
2 teaspoons baking powder
1 teaspoon baking soda
2 organic brown eggs
¾ cup buttermilk
½ cup organic unfiltered apple juice
½ cup rolled oats
1½ cups Granny Smith apples, cored, peeled, chopped
½ cup walnuts, chopped (optional)

FOR THE FROSTING

¼ cup maple syrup (Crown Maple, very dark color, strong taste)
1 tablespoon European-style butter
1 capful pure vanilla extract
1 cup confectioners' sugar
Apple slices for garnish

In a mixing bowl, combine flour, sugar, baking powder, and baking soda. Add eggs, beaten, buttermilk, and apple juice. Stir well. Add oats. Fold in apples and nuts. Use a ¼-cup ice cream scoop or spoon and place batter into a cupcake tin lined with cupcake papers. Bake at 400 degrees F approximately 20 minutes or until light golden brown and firm to touch. Cool. Top with frosting. Sprinkle with nuts and garnish with fresh apple slices.

For the frosting, combine syrup and butter, melted. Add sugar.and extract (You may add more if you like a thick frosting; for a creamier consistency, use more syrup.) Place one small circle of frosting on top of each muffin, flattened for a nice round look. Top with nuts if preferred.

Avocado Coconut Bowl with Pistachio-Coconut Granola and Fresh Juice

Power bowls are easy to make and super nutritious. Spa goers enjoy this superfood breakfast bowl, and for good reason. Enjoy the flavors and textures. You'll likely get a boost of energy to help you get a move on in the morning.

FOR THE BOWL

1 avocado
¼ cup orange juice
½ cup coconut milk
½ banana
¼ cup blueberries for garnish
¼ cup strawberries, sliced, for garnish

FOR THE GRANOLA

1 whole banana (or 2 halves)
2 teaspoons cinnamon

1 cup honey
1½ cups maple syrup
¼ cup coconut oil
1 bag (32 ounces) organic rolled oats
1½ boxes (10 ounces each) brown rice cereal
½ teaspoon salt
8 cups coconut flakes
4 cups toasted pistachios

In a blender or food processor, mix avocado, juice, milk, and banana. Pour mixture into bowls. Add berries on top. Refrigerate.

For the granola, heat the oven to 250 degrees F. Combine the banana, cinnamon, honey, maple syrup, and oil in a blender. Place this mixture into a large bowl with oats, cereal, salt, coconut flakes, and pistachios. Toss the ingredients together to combine and thoroughly mix. Spread evenly onto six large sheet pans and bake 20 minutes. Repeat this process three times for 60 minutes total. The mixture should be slightly crispy. Remove and set on a rack to cool for 1 hour before putting into airtight container.

½ cup of the fruit is an average serving. The granola yields a lot, so it's difficult to give an exact servings count.

(Courtesy: Chef Curtis Cooke, Cal-a-Vie Health Spa)

Blueberry Pancakes with Vermont Maple Syrup and Herbal Tea

When I traveled three thousand miles from California to Montreal, Quebec, I had planned to experience a breakfast-in-bed fantasy. In the morning, I'd awake and order room service superfoods: blueberry pancakes with maple syrup and a carafe of coffee. But due to a late arrival and jet lag, I awoke at noon, and the menu options had changed. My first meal ended up being a comfort superfood pick of grilled cheese with tomatoes on whole-wheat bread, even though blueberry pancakes with maple syrup were on my mind.

1½ cups whole-wheat flour (King Arthur)
¼ cup sugar
1 tablespoon baking powder
½ teaspoon baking soda
½ teaspoon sea salt
1 teaspoon ground cinnamon
1 teaspoon pure vanilla extract
¾ cup half-and-half
¾ cup buttermilk
2 eggs
2 cups blueberries (save half for topping pancakes)
1–2 tablespoons unsalted butter for greasing frying pan
½ cup sliced almonds
Maple syrup (Crown Maple)

In a mixing bowl, combine the dry ingredients (flour, sugar, baking powder, baking soda, salt, spice) and extract. Add half-and-half, buttermilk and eggs. Stir. Fold in 1 cup of blueberries. Lightly butter a frying pan over medium heat. Drop the batter by ½ cups onto the pan and spread into round circles. Cook the pancakes a few minutes. Turn the pancakes over and cook 1–2 more minutes. Repeat with the remaining pancake batter. Serve the pancakes with the rest of the blueberries, almonds, and maple syrup.

Makes 3–4 servings.

Citrus Muffins with a Twist and English Breakfast Tea

Welcome to my breakfast muffin recipe. I recall awakening early in the morning. My mission was to go to Sacramento to pick up a new addition to my family. Not a big breakfast person, I stopped en route at a convenience store and purchased a packaged muffin. While it stopped my stomach from growling, a home-baked muffin would have been, well, special on this trip. Upon my arrival, an elderly woman who lived on the ranch handed me a wake-up gift. "How adorable," I exclaimed. My arms wrapped around a twelve-pound fur ball—a ten-week-old Australian shepherd puppy complete with puppy breath. And we traveled back home to Lake Tahoe to begin a new life. A few years later, I made lemon muffins late at night. In the morning, I brewed a cup of coffee and warmed up a fresh muffin. I took the two treats back to bed. Turning on the TV for *CBS This Morning*, I looked to the right of me. A full-grown Aussie with amber eyes met my eyes. It was a superfood breakfast with my super puppy with big, fluffy paws.

1 large orange (cut in half and use ½ cup juice)
½ cup organic 2-percent milk
½ cup European-style butter (melted)
¼ cup sugar
1 large brown egg
1 capful pure vanilla extract
1¾ cup whole-wheat self-rising flour (King Arthur)
2–3 teaspoons lemon rind
Raw sugar
Mint leaves for garnish

In a large bowl, stir together juice and milk. Add butter, sugar, egg, and extract, stir well. Add flour (sift or whisk fine with a fork) and lemon rind until smooth, without lumps. Fill muffin cups with batter. (Use a ½-cup ice cream scoop to make muffins the same size.) Bake 20 minutes or until tops are light golden brown and firm to touch. Cool and remove from pan. Sprinkle muffin tops with sugar. Garnish with mint. You can remove muffin wrappers for a nicer look. Breakfast muffins store well in an airtight container.

Makes 10 muffins.

Greek Yogurt, Granola, and Seasonal Fresh Berries and Black Tea

One morning in Montreal, Quebec, I did order this sweet and simple breakfast. It took me back in time to when I was a grad student at San Francisco State University. I left the campus to visit a café nearby. When I was served plain, thick creamy yogurt, fresh fruit, and honey, it was a turning point, telling me to forego flavored yogurts and savor superfoods as is. Also, eating yogurt and berries filled the void for my bout of homesickness.

2 cups plain Greek yogurt
1 cup fresh strawberries, sliced
1 cup granola
Honey

In a parfait glass, layer yogurt, granola, and berries. Drizzle honey on top. Serve with black tea and lemon slices.

Makes 2 servings.

Super Smoothies Bar

Smoothies—savory and sweet types—are sprinkled throughout the end chapters of *The Healing Powers of Superfoods*. But here are several more nutritious and energizing smoothies that deserve sharing and whipping up. But sabotaging these beverages with exotic scoops of rice protein and goji berries isn't going to be found here. The ingredients I use are easily found at your supermarket.

Once when I was window-shopping up and down the streets in Palo Alto, California, I stopped at a progressive ice cream shop complete with smoothies. The girl at the counter asked me, "What type of protein powder?" I shook my head and answered, "None." She proceeded with her array of milk choices, including almond, coconut, and goat. I scrunched my nose and shook my head, saying, "No. Just normal." I ended up with a strawberry smoothie that included fresh berries, natural juice, honey, and crushed iced. And this basic smoothie, instead of one with strange stuff that I can't pronounce, was delightful.

So, welcome to the real superfood drinks (without bizarre eats like on a *Fear Factor* TV episode). My super creamy, coffee-infused Mocha Wake-Up Smoothie and decadent, thick Double Chocolate Shake/ Smoothie are two of my personal favorites, inspired by my past as a college student and kid. Thanks to the old-fashioned, classic superfoods (including fruit, ice, ice cream, and nut butter), you'll get super nutrients and super flavor and super creamy texture.

There is a wide world of superfoods to put into your smoothies (cold or hot)—all with nutritional virtues that'll boost your mood, increase alertness, enhance energy, aid in weight loss, and even add years to your life because you're getting a lot of antiaging superfoods blended into one drink.

Apple Nut Smoothie (Hot)
Double Chocolate Shake/Smoothie
Mocha Wake-Up Smoothie
Pumpkin Spice Smoothie (Hot)
Raspberry-Basil Smoothie

Apple Nut Smoothie (Hot)

❖ ❖ ❖

Smoothies are known and savored from their cold first sip to the last, thanks to ice, which is often used to keep them chilled and creamy. Hot smoothies are comforting and nutritious, too, much like a cup of soup. An Apple Nut Smoothie can be enjoyed chilled, but on a chilly day, especially in the fall, a hot one is like a hot apple cider, but thicker and more comforting. It is similar to a cold smoothie or milkshake, but heating it up makes the smoothie, well, hot—and something every smoothie lover must give a try.

On a late fall Sunday afternoon, I instinctively wanted to go to the local resort casino and play the slot machines because I sensed it was a lucky day. Sitting at the one-dollar slots, I played the game but was envious of the machine next to me. Soon, the man playing it left, leaving the slot machine I had bonded with vacant. After a couple of spins I hit the numbers: $2,000. It was an exciting moment, and once back home, I celebrated by creating a hot apple nut smoothie inspired by the feel-good-day win.

1 cup Honeycrisp or Fuji apples, chopped (leave the peels on)
½ cup unsweetened apple juice
½ cup fresh orange juice
2 tablespoons walnuts
½ teaspoon cinnamon
1 cup ice cubes
Vanilla Greek yogurt or ice cream for garnish
Mint leaves for garnish
Cinnamon sticks (grind and use as topping)

Put all ingredients, including apples, juices, nuts, cinnamon, and ice cubes, in a blender. Mix until smooth. Pour apple mixture into a saucepan. Warm until hot. Pour into mugs. Top with yogurt, mint, and ground cinnamon sticks.

Makes 2 servings.

Double Chocolate Shake/Smoothie

This decadent drink is a creation of milk, ice cream, and flavorings such as chocolate syrup. Back in my waitressing days (yes, I was a server), I'd make milkshakes, which took time, using steel containers full of ingredients that you'd stick into a machine to get "shaked." (My shakes often whirled too fast, spilling onto the floor, which ended my server days.) Milkshakes were messy to make and usually included imitation vanilla ice cream. No fresh fruits, seeds, or nuts. But times have changed, or maybe I continue to think outside of the can and shake things up so that my shakes are whole and natural.

When I penned *The Healing Powers of Chocolate*, I was treated at a European-style hotel spa in Reno. Imagine savoring a Chocolate Silk Hydrotherapy Bath in an oversized claw-foot Jacuzzi-style bathtub full of bubbling water and a chocolate scent while savoring house-made chocolate truffles. After thirty minutes, there was more to enjoy in chocolate heaven. I was given a chocolate scrub/French manicure and a tall chocolate milkshake to sip. But the perfectionist in me now says, "The shake could have been dark chocolate infused with fresh fruit chunks for a healthier kick." So, just for you, dear readers, I've concocted an awesome chocolate delight that'll wow your eyes and taste buds—right at home.

½ cup organic half-and-half
¼ cup organic low-fat milk
1 cup premium, all-natural chocolate ice cream
1 teaspoon premium unsweetened cocoa powder
½ cup banana slices
1 tablespoon nut butter (your choice)
4–5 ice cubes
Strawberries and nuts for topping and/or garnish

Put all ingredients including half-and-half, milk, ice cream, cocoa powder, banana, nut butter, and ice, in a blender. If it has a "smoothie" button on it, all the better. Blend until thick, but not too thin. Pour into glass mugs or glasses. Garnish with berries and/or nuts. Hold the whipped cream unless it's the real stuff you whip up yourself from scratch. You can put the chocolate shake/smoothies in the freezer for 15–20 minutes to make them colder.

Makes 2 small shakes or 1 large one.

Mocha Wake-Up Smoothie

This smoothie was a super cool treat one week during a Lake Tahoe heat wave in the late summer. The chocolate is calming and energizing, and the healthful ingredients are flavorful and, well, summer-healthy. It has a nostalgic Dairy Queen frosty flavor to it, but with a twenty-first-century dark(er) chocolaty taste. A homemade smoothie is simple to create, and as I always say, you can control the ingredients to keep it healthy, just the way *you* like it.

½ cup all-natural coffee–chocolate chip gelato
½ cup all-natural vanilla bean gelato
½ cup low-fat organic milk
¼ cup cinnamon-flavored premium coffee, brewed, cold
2 tablespoons walnuts, finely chopped
2 tablespoons chocolate hazelnut butter (Nutella)
Cinnamon stick for garnish

Combine gelatos, milk, coffee, walnuts, and nut butter in a blender. Set on "smoothie" or blend until thick and creamy. Pour into a mug and add cinnamon stick and a straw.

Makes 1 serving.

Pumpkin Spice Smoothie (Hot)

❖ ❖ ❖

During autumn, pumpkin love is part of the season. One fall day, I wanted something warm to savor for Indian summer. Instead of a slice of cold pumpkin pie or pumpkin fudge, I whipped up a hot pumpkin smoothie with a superfoods touch. Pumpkin is a touted superfood, but so are gelato and pumpkin seeds.

½ cup all-natural pumpkin ice cream or gelato (homemade or
   premium store-bought)
½ cup low-fat organic milk
½ cup pumpkin (puree, canned)
1 tablespoon pumpkin spice
½ cup ice cubes
Whipped cream for garnish
Cinnamon or cocoa powder for garnish
Shelled pumpkin seeds for garnish

Combine ice cream or gelato, milk, pumpkin, spice, and ice in blender. Blend until smooth. Place pumpkin mixture into a saucepan. Heat until hot. Pour into a mug. Top with whipped cream. Sprinkle with cinnamon or cocoa powder. Top with seeds.

Makes 1 serving.

Raspberry-Basil Smoothie

Blueberries are a popular superfood. as I noted when sharing my love for other berries. In the summertime, berries are plentiful and fresh. As a kid, I recall picking wild raspberries in my friend's backyard. They were sweet and tart as well as delicious on a hot afternoon. This smoothie, inspired by my life in the calming suburbs, takes me back in time to when life was a time of play and clocks were ignored.

½ cup plain Greek yogurt
½ cup low-fat organic almond milk
½ fresh orange juice
1 cup fresh or frozen raspberries
2 tablespoons fresh basil, chopped
2 tablespoons nut butter (Nutella)
Cinnamon stick and fresh mint for garnish

Combine yogurt, milk, juice, berries, basil, and nut butter in a blender. Set on "smoothie" or blend until thick and creamy. Pour into a mug and add cinnamon stick and a straw.

Makes 2 servings.

Superfoods-Infused Assorted Appetizers

There's a good vibe when you are creating fresh appetizers, also called hors d'oeuvres and canapés. Appetizers are served up at posh hotels in the late afternoons and before dinners—and they can be good for you. Royal Heirloom Tomato Bruschetta and Super-Duper Cheesy Potato Skins, for instance, are full of antioxidants to help boost your immune system and potatoes and cheese, rich in potassium and calcium, are bloat-busting and calming comfort food cuties.

Appetizers can be delicious and healthful using superfoods. For example, the Spinach-Yogurt Dip Bread Bowl boasts plenty of nutrients, and accompanied with raw vegetables like fresh broccoli, cauliflower florets, and cherry tomatoes, this hors d'oeuvre can almost be a light and ultrasatisfying dinner.

Spinach-Yogurt Dip Bread Bowl
Super Fresh Shellfish Cocktail
Roasted Whole Cauliflower
Royal Heirloom Tomato Bruschetta
Super-Duper Cheesy Potato Skins

Spinach-Yogurt Dip Bread Bowl

The days of onion dip made with dried soup mix and served with potato chips were from the twentieth century. Switching it up to a fresh, eye-catching dip bread bowl is something to write home to mom about—and she may just love it. I'm talking superfoods: spinach, Greek yogurt, cheese, artisanal whole-grain bread and crackers, and cruciferous vegetables. This recipe is inspired by my love for superfoods and for finger food gone wild and yummy!

½ cup cream cheese, softened
½ cup mayonnaise with olive oil
½ cup plain Greek yogurt
1 teaspoon scallions, chopped
1 cup fresh spinach, chopped, dry
2 tablespoons parsley
½ cup mild white cheddar, shredded
Sea salt and ground pepper, to taste
1 round loaf artisanal whole-grain sourdough bread
1 tablespoon extra-virgin olive oil or European-style butter
½ cup Parmesan, shavings
Whole-grain crackers
Raw cruciferous vegetables

In a mixing bowl, combine cream cheese, mayonnaise, yogurt, and scallions. Stir until smooth. Add spinach, parsley, cheddar, salt, and pepper. Chill in refrigerator. Meanwhile, slice the top off the bread. With a knife, cut out the bread to make a bowl. Set the cut-out pieces of bread aside to cut into squares later. Put the chilled cheese-spinach mixture into the bread bowl. Brush bowl with olive oil or melted butter. Top with Parmesan. Bake at 400 degrees F about 30 minutes or until bubbly and golden brown. Serve with artisanal whole-grain crackers, bread squares, and raw cruciferous vegetables. You can also serve this dish cold—no baking needed.

Super Fresh Shellfish Cocktail

California offers the luxury of eating by rivers, lakes, and oceans, like at Fisherman's Wharf and on the San Francisco Peninsula, which is dotted with waterfront eateries. Shrimp cocktail was a favorite of mine, but then I turned to crab. Now, older and wiser, I'm thinking, "Why not make a minicombo?" Shellfish is delicious on the coast because you get it fresh. This simple recipe, complete with California avocados, lemons, tomatoes, and shellfish, is West Coast-inspired.

1 cup each fresh crabmeat and shrimp, cooked
2 Roma tomatoes, chopped
1 scallion, chopped fine
⅓ cup extra-virgin olive oil
¼ cup fresh basil, chopped
¼ cup fresh lemon juice
Sea salt and ground pepper, to taste
½ avocado, chopped
2 eggs, boiled, sliced
Whole-grain bread, sliced
Extra-virgin olive oil, in a small bowl

In a mixing bowl, combine shellfish, tomatoes, scallion, olive oil, basil, and lemon juice. Add salt and pepper. Top with avocado cubes and egg slices. Serve with artisanal whole-grain bread dipped in olive oil.

Makes 3–4 servings.

Roasted Whole Cauliflower

❖ ❖ ❖

Whole roasted cauliflower has been appearing on trendy restaurant menus and even the Food Network channel. Gorgeously crusted on the outside and tender on the inside, this visually striking preparation of cauliflower is popular among chefs for a host of reasons: It's budget friendly, ridiculously simple to make, and guaranteed to impress guests, either as a main dish or on the side.

This dish has become a modern classic as chefs around the world are working out new ways to push vegetables into the center of the plate.

One head of cauliflower
½ cup extra-virgin olive oil
Kosher salt

Preheat the oven to 375 degrees F and place a rack in the middle position. Wash and dry the cauliflower head. Remove the leaves. Flip it over and remove the stem by cutting a cone into the bottom of the cauliflower with a paring knife. Do not remove too much of the stem or the florets will start to separate. Rub all over with olive oil and salt. Be generous with both! Place the cauliflower in a cast-iron frying pan or an ovenproof dish. Cover with aluminum foil to retain the heat and steam. Cook for 30 minutes, covered. After 30 minutes, remove the foil, drizzle with more olive oil, and roast for 1 hour. Test for doneness by piercing it with a knife. You should not meet any resistance. Remove when the cauliflower is nicely browned on the outside. Transfer to a dish and drizzle with more olive oil to finish. To serve, carve the cauliflower into wedges at the table.

(Courtesy: North American Olive Oil Association,
www.aboutoliveoil.com)

Royal Heirloom Tomato Bruschetta

Meet a sophisticated Italian appetizer called crostini or bruschetta. These versatile cuties are made with small slices of toasted bread and an assortment of toppings. Think cheeses, vegetables, herbs, and even fruit. These scrumptious treats go back centuries and were served by peasants who didn't have plates, but these days crostini can be served to all classes of people—rich, poor, and in-between.

On my summer trip to Victoria, British Columbia, I was one of the lucky chosen few (a treat to the suite guests) to enjoy the concierge dining room's appetizer bar. At 5:00 P.M., I entered the highest floor of the hotel, with its picturesque panoramic view of the boat harbor, into a room complete with special food for special people. As a finicky semivegetarian, my attention was won by the crackers, cheeses, and olives—not the cooked bean dish or mystery meat in a metal container. I scooped up a plate full of the edibles and fled back to my room, with its own million-dollar Inner Harbour view. I placed different foods on the assortment of crackers and pretended they were the classic bruschetta appetizers. Here they are again, Victoria-inspired with a taste of Tahoe.

4 slices of a baguette or French bread (toasted or warmed up in the
    microwave) or multigrain herb crackers
4 cubes or slices of cheese (cheddar or goat)
2 heirloom or Roma Tomatoes, chopped or sliced
Several olives, pitted, sliced
Red onion, chopped (optional)

Top each piece of bread or cracker with cheese, tomato, olives, and onion. Heat up or serve cold.

These tasty appetizers are one of my favorite superfood pairings when time is not on my side. They're quick and easy to put together, filling and fun to eat, and easy on the eyes. What's not to love? These crunchy cheese-tomato cuties can be brunch or a snack and even a light dinner.

Super-Duper Cheesy Potato Skins

❖ ❖ ❖

These potato skins take me back to the nineties, when I'd go to a TGI Friday's restaurant and place an order on nights out with the girls. Cheesy, gooey, and hot taters made the night exciting. Now, I make them at home for fun. Serving these gems with hot or iced tea (or your chilled brew of choice), flavored water, or a glass of red or white wine makes any season memorable, whether you're enjoying the hot stuff with a mate or solo. Either way it's all good, and this appetizer is a favorite for both men and women (of all ages). Caveat: You can make a potato skins bar like a baked potato bar. Put out different bites and bits of superfood toppings, including chicken and turkey, Greek yogurt, crucifers, kale, spinach, and tomatoes. Let people have fun building their own potato skins!

4 medium russet potatoes
2–4 tablespoons European-style butter
Dash of sea salt
Ground black pepper, to taste
1½ cups Monterey Jack and sharp cheddar, shredded
2 tablespoons kale, chopped
2 tablespoons green onions, chopped (optional)
¼ cup each, Greek yogurt and sour cream

Preheat oven to 350 degrees F. Wash potatoes. Prick each one with a fork and bake about 1 hour. Cool. Cut potatoes in half lengthwise. Scoop out flesh, leaving shells. Place shells into deep baking dish. Melt butter and drizzle it over the skins. Sprinkle with salt and pepper. Put skins into oven, turned up to 375 degrees F. Bake about 10 minutes, remove. Turn potatoes over and heat another 10 minutes or until brown and crispy. Place potato skins upright and pile on the cheese. Bake a few more minutes. Remove. Top with fresh kale and onion. Serve hot with a small dish of yogurt or sour cream.

Makes 3–4 servings.

Tater tips: Cool the potatoes before scooping out the flesh. Use a knife or spoon to gently cut a rectangle of potato about ½ inch wide to use for the skins to look like an open boat shape. Olive oil mixed with butter is an option, but butter makes the potato skins super crispy. Onions, salt, and pepper give the potato skins extra flavor. Cooked, crispy bacon bits are a must-have for meat lovers, but you can substitute the sea vegetable dulse for the same texture. And chopped tomatoes, parsley, and/or chives are great for vegetarians.

Superfoods-Infused Salads

Vegetable platters, which can include broccoli and cauliflower, or artisanal cheese plates with gouda and cheddar cheeses, apple slices, and whole-grain breads (with seeds and nuts) are all super delicious and filling. Classic salads such as cobb salad, chef's salad, and a basic tossed green salad as sides and entrees are tasty and good for you, and even better with whole-grain artisanal bread.

Adding cruciferous vegetables, such as kale and spinach, and seasonal fruits (or dried berries and nuts) can give you "so good!" moments to be enjoyed at home or while traveling. An entrée salad (cold or hot) or side salad for brunch, a light dinner, or a snack any time of the day is healthful year-round.

The idea of three big square meals a day was a twentieth-century style; nowadays grazing on salads as minimeals or main meals is accepted as a healthier way to get your superfoods. Super Healthy Crucifer-Shrimp Salad is a great way to get your fill of cruciferous vegetables, leafy greens, shellfish, and tomatoes. Tossed Salad with Hiziki (Sea Vegetable) and Italian Dressing is mixing it up with the old and new ingredients and local produce from garden to table, making this dish an exotic delight with traditional roots.

Super Healthy Crucifer-Shrimp Salad
California Egg-Potato Salad
Harvest Greens and Vinaigrette
Tossed Salad with Hiziki (Sea Vegetable)
and Italian Dressing

Super Healthy Crucifer-Shrimp Salad

❖ ❖ ❖

1 cup broccoli, cut into florets
1 cup cauliflower, cut into florets
6 ounces water-packed shrimp, cooked
½ cup cherry tomatoes, sliced in half
Sea salt and pepper, to taste
¼ cup basil, chopped
¼ cup fresh lemon juice
4 teaspoons extra-virgin olive oil
1 teaspoon red wine vinegar

In a pan, steam the broccoli and cauliflower until tender crisp. Put them in a shallow serving bowl and add the shrimp, tomatoes, salt, pepper, and basil. Pour lemon juice, olive oil, and vinegar over the mixture, toss gently. (Use more or less for your preference.) Keep refrigerated until ready to serve.

Makes 3–4 cups.

California Egg-Potato Salad

During the Great Recession of 2008, it was like going back to grad school days for me; I was rolling pennies to pay for store runs. Images of the characters from *The Grapes of Wrath* came to mind when I'd go to the supermarket. One day at our friendly Safeway, I grabbed a bag of potatoes. (Single ones are nicer, but bulk is more budget friendly.) But it was at that time I became resourceful and made eating on the cheap healthy and flavorful. So, here is a revised recipe inspired by my mom but with a new, improved West Coast twist.

4 russet, yellow or red, potatoes, washed and boiled (with skins on)
2 hard-boiled organic brown eggs, chopped
¾ cup mayonnaise with olive oil dressing (store bought)
½ cup green bell pepper, chopped
2 tablespoons red onion, chopped
Black pepper and sea salt, to taste
1 cup baby spinach, chopped
¼ cup almonds, sliced
½ cup blue cheese, crumbled
4 Roma or cherry tomatoes, sliced, for garnish.

Cut potatoes into cubes (leave skins on) and place them into a large mixing bowl. Add eggs and mayonnaise, and mix well. Add bell pepper, onion, pepper, and salt. Chill in refrigerator. Serve a large scoop of potato salad on a bed of spinach leaves. Top with almonds and cheese. Garnish with tomato.

Makes 4–6 servings.

Harvest Greens and Vinaigrette

❖ ❖ ❖

If you live in a region where autumn weather includes warm Indian summer days and chilly prewinter nights, then you know how the change can play games with your appetite. It's best to go with the flow and enter the seasonal change slowly with hot and cold superfoods so you keep your sanity! This is a Lake Tahoe/Sierra-inspired greens, nuts, and berries salad, complete with a hot beverage for fall.

FOR THE DRESSING

½ cup olive oil
3 tablespoons red wine vinegar
½ teaspoon Dijon mustard
Honey (use sparingly, to taste)
Dash of pepper

FOR THE SALAD

1 cup kale, chopped
1 cup baby spinach, chopped
¼ cup walnuts, chopped
½ cup fresh berries (cranberries—yes! They're tart but good.)
Red onion, sliced thin (about 2 tablespoons, optional)
Parmesan, shaved or shredded
½ cup chicken or shrimp (cooked, chopped)

Mix olive oil, vinegar, mustard, honey, and pepper for dressing. Chill in fridge. In a bowl, combine greens, nuts, berries, onion, cheese, and chicken or shrimp. Put in refrigerator. Whisk up dressing and drizzle over your salad mixture.

Pair your greens with a mug of hot apple cider with a cinnamon stick. Or brew a cup of cinnamon- or vanilla-flavored coffee, add organic low-fat milk, and if you really want a treat, put on a dollop of whipped cream and sprinkle it with pumpkin pie spice or cocoa powder.

Makes 1–2 servings.

Tossed Salad with Hiziki (Sea Vegetable) and Italian Dressing

❖ ❖ ❖

Sea vegetables and I have a history, as you know by now. I've discovered if you use less rather than more and pair this different superfood with superfoods you love, it can work wonders. You won't be tempted to stash the sea monster, but will willingly (almost) eat it and maybe get an awareness that you like it!

FOR THE SALAD

2 tablespoons hiziki, washed, soaked 15 minutes in warm water, drained (Eden)
2 cups mixed baby salad greens or lettuce
1 medium tomato, sliced
¼ cup carrots, coarsely grated
1 avocado, seeded, peeled, and sliced or cubed

FOR THE DRESSING

¼ cup extra-virgin olive oil (Eden)
½ cup water
2 tablespoons red wine vinegar (Eden)
2 tablespoons organic maple syrup
1½ tablespoons shoyu soy sauce (Eden)
1 teaspoon dried basil
½ teaspoon dried oregano
2 cloves garlic, minced
⅛ teaspoon paprika powder
¼ teaspoon freshly ground pepper
2 tablespoons fresh parsley

Place the hiziki in a small saucepan, add cold water to just cover the hiziki. Cover the pan and bring to a boil. Reduce the flame and simmer 10 minutes. Pour the hiziki into a strainer and rinse under cold water. Place the hiziki into a salad bowl with the salad greens, tomato, carrot and avocado. Toss to mix. Put in refrigerator. Prepare the dressing by placing all ingredients in a blender. Pulse several seconds to blend evenly. Place the dressing in a serving container. Pour over salad before serving.

(Courtesy: Eden Foods)

Assorted Soups and Sandwiches

As a kid, soup was lunch or dinner and touted for its soothing benefits if I was hit by the flu or cold. Also, at fancy restaurants, the soup of the day was offered before the entrée, where I usually opted for a salad. Nowadays, chunky soups and comforting chowders are not only popular for feeding a crowd, I'm on the bandwagon, too—*if* they're homemade and superfoods are part of the soup.

Using organic broth, superfoods such as fresh vegetables, and whole-grain pasta, you can make a bowl of Bone Broth Vegetable Potpourri Soup or Fresh Tomato Soup that is filling and super delicious. Pairing a hot soup with fresh, warm, whole-grain artisanal bread (spread with butter or dipped in olive oil) is how I do twenty-first-century soup, and yes, soups are no longer for the sick or just filler for fancy dining.

Bone Broth Vegetable Potpourri Soup
Fresh Tomato Soup
Dulse Miso Soup
Goat Cheese Panini
Grilled Cheese with Tomatoes

Bone Broth Vegetable Potpourri Soup

As a self-professed hypochondriac, after hearing all the doom-and-gloom virus reports for 2018, I thought a cold was paying me a visit. On the upside, the weather was good, so without snow to shovel or crackling fires to make, not to forget walking the dog on black ice, I decided to prepare. Water, lemon juice, vegetables, herbs, and tea were stocked and ready for me to be "woman down." During a three day holiday, I escaped to the bed. My refuge included clean flannel sheets with cozy comforters, two companion animals, one log into the fireplace (with the promise to burn $4\frac{1}{2}$ hours), the popular TV mini-series *Big Little Lies*—and tea. On day two, I was surprised. After making soup and drinking tea—no cold, no flu. I survived. So, here's the recipe to fight a cold that may be coming to visit you.

1 carton (32 ounces) organic low-sodium chicken bone broth (Pacific)
¼ cup red or yellow onion, chopped
2 tablespoons fresh garlic, minced
½ cup celery, chopped
¼ cup fresh basil, chopped
2 tablespoons Italian seasoning
2 large Roma tomatoes, chopped
½ cup carrots and cauliflower, chopped
1–1½ cups whole-grain spaghetti
1 cup whole-grain pasta shells
Sea salt and ground pepper, to taste
¼ cup fresh shredded Parmesan for garnish

Pour broth into a large pot. Bring to a boil. Heat water in another pan, and boil onion, garlic, celery, basil, seasoning, tomatoes, carrots, and cauliflower until tender. Drain and place in broth. Simmer 15 minutes. In another pot, boil pasta for several minutes until cooked. Add pasta and salt and pepper to soup mixture. Simmer about 10 minutes. Top with cheese. Serve with slices of local artisanal sourdough French whole-grain bread spread with real butter.

Makes 6 servings.

This easy-to-make vegetable soup tastes much better than the stuff from a can. The scent of garlic and onion fills the kitchen, and it feels like you've been cooking home-style soup all day. Pairing a bowl of hot soup with a slice of fresh, warm bread will warm you up and give you that warm and fuzzy feeling, too.

Not to forget, brew a pot of premium black or herbal tea—another superfood that is a must-have in your diet regime. Use tea bags or leaves. Add fresh lemon and local honey—two more good-for-you foods to boost your immune system. Sipping tea before and after this meal adds good-for-you disease-fighting antioxidants. And they, my friends, will help you keep the colds and flu at bay. Is it worth the trouble to cook up a batch of DIY soup and brew a tea potion? You bet, especially if you want to be ready for the next storm.

Fresh Tomato Soup

❖ ❖ ❖

I remember, when I was a child, Campbell's canned tomato soup was dished up with a tuna sandwich for lunch. I liked chicken noodle soup and vegetable soup, but the red stuff in the bowl? I played with it. Adding oyster crackers just made my childhood games more creative; the add-on wasn't enough incentive to eat the tomato glop.

Now, I know it wasn't the tomato variety I turned my nose up at, it was the way it was prepared. After all, I love tomato-based soups with chicken and fish. So, this Fresh Tomato Soup reminds me of those; it's garden-fresh and paired with fresh, warm French bread, so it's a keeper without a can.

¼ cup Marsala olive fruit oil
4 garlic cloves, chopped
¼ cup onions, thinly sliced (optional)
3 tablespoons flour
1 cup sherry or white wine
2 pounds fresh tomatoes, peeled, diced
4 cups chicken broth
¼ cup fresh basil or parsley, chopped
Salt, pepper, and cayenne, to taste
2 bay leaves
1 teaspoon celery seeds, ground
2 cups croutons
Romano, grated, or mozzarella, shredded
Celery leaves

In a Dutch oven, over medium heat, add oil and garlic, cook until soft. (If you choose to use onions, add after garlic.) Stir in flour, cook until smooth. Add wine, simmer a few minutes. Add tomatoes, broth, basil or parsley, salt, pepper, cayenne, bay leaves, and celery seeds, cover and simmer 20–30 minutes. Remove bay leaves before serving. Serve with cheese and croutons. Garnish with celery leaves (center part).

Makes 4–6 servings.

(Courtesy: Gemma Sanita Sciabica, from *Cooking with California Olive Oil: Treasured Family Recipes*)

Dulse Miso Soup

❖ ❖ ❖

The most exotic superfood choice in this book is sea vegetables. Since they do contain compounds that have healing powers, it seems fair to include some recipes, like this soup, that may change both my mind and yours about eating a different superfood. A small bowl of hot Dulse Miso Soup with whole-grain bread may find its way into your home, especially for the health-conscious folks or foodies looking for something new.

4 cups water
¼ cup Bonito Flakes, crushed into small pieces (optional) (Eden)
¼ cup onions, thinly sliced
¼ cup carrots, julienned
¼ cup fresh green beans, sliced in 1½-inch lengths
½ pound organic tofu, cubed
⅓ cup shiro miso, or to taste (Eden)
2 tablespoons whole leaf dulse, soaked 5 minutes in cold water,
    chopped (Eden)
2 tablespoons green onions, thinly sliced, for garnish

Place water in saucepan and bring to boil. Add Bonito Flakes and onions. Reduce the flame to medium-low and cook 2–3 minutes. Add carrots and green beans, cover, and simmer 4–5 minutes. Reduce the flame to low. Add the tofu, miso, and dulse. Cook 2 minutes. Serve garnished with green onion.

[Assuming one cup is a normal size serving for soup, this recipe makes approximately 4 servings.]

(Courtesy: Eden Foods)

Goat Cheese Panini

One chilly afternoon after viewing the movie *It's Complicated*, I made my first panini inspired by Meryl Streep's film dish, a hot cheesy French sandwich called croque monsieur. It wowed and wooed the male characters played by Steve Martin and Alec Baldwin—and me. It's a simple sandwich with an egg base, ham, tomato, cheese, and bread—one or two slices. I chose to go the Italian panini route—no eggs or ham. So this is my version of a cheese panini full of deliciousness. And for the record, I did not choose smoked goat cheese.

2–3 tablespoons olive oil or European-style butter
4 thick slices whole-grain organic European-style French bread (or a
    baguette)
3 slices mozzarella
2 tablespoons crumbled goat cheese
1 Roma tomato, sliced
2 tablespoons fresh basil, chopped

On medium heat, use a large skillet to add oil or butter, melt, and add bread. Top two slices of the bread with cheeses and tomato. Then cover them with the other two slices of buttered or oiled bread. Place another smaller pan (or spatula) on top of sandwiches. Cook 3–5 minutes on each side or until brown. Slice each hot sandwich in half. Top with fresh basil.

You can also use the oven broiler. A Panini press or grill is nice to achieve grill marks, but two skillets or an oven broiler can achieve the toasted grill imprint, sort of. The crunch of the soft but crispy bread and the gooeyness of the cheese are, well, good (especially if you use premium ingredients).

Makes 2 servings.

Grilled Cheese with Tomatoes

I've dished out kudos to the grilled cheese sandwich time after time. Actually, I've become the grilled cheese queen of this comfort food sandwich. If put together the right way—my way—this simple classic can become a gourmet delight. When traveling, I always order this sandwich, whether it's in Montreal, Quebec, or Seattle, Washington. My order calls for a variety of superfoods: whole-grain bread, cheddar or Monterey jack (or both), fresh tomatoes, and cut in half. This sandwich is inspired by my childhood, but it's a grown-up version with Mediterranean finesse.

Olive oil or European-style butter (enough to coat the pan)
2 slices cheddar
2 slices mozzarella
2 slices Monterey Jack or Gouda
4 thick slices whole-grain bread
1 large tomato, off the vine, sliced
Ground pepper and sea salt, to taste
Basil or parsley for garnish

In a skillet, on medium heat, heat up oil or butter. Place cheese slices on 2 pieces of bread, add tomato slices. Add pepper and salt. Cover each slice of bread with another slice. Let both sandwiches cook 4–5 minutes or until the bottom is golden brown. Flip and repeat. Remove from stovetop. Slice in half, top with basil or parsley, and serve hot with a bowl of soup.

Makes 2 servings.

Pasta Plates

Whole-grain pasta is a versatile superfood and not to be left out of your daily diet. Pasta comes in all shapes and sizes. Paired with other superfoods, including leafy greens, crucifers, cheese, and tomatoes, it's like a crescendo in a film or music. Pasta plates with superfoods are often found on menus at restaurants.

Twentieth-century classic pasta dishes include macaroni and cheese (a favorite of kids) and linguini and clams (a must-have dish for fish and pasta lovers). These recipes can be cooked up, then dished up with a fresh twist on superfoods. Use whole-grain pasta and the healthiest cheese with tomatoes for mac and cheese and fresh clams and lemon for linguini and clams for a wholesome and creative new spin on favorite foods. Mixing it up is not only fun, it also is a nice refreshing change for the palate (at any age). Pasta dishes can work year-round with the aid of super superfoods.

Pasta Power Bowl with Superfoods
Linguine with Clam Sauce
Lobster Mac and Cheese
Noodle Salad with Sesame Dressing
Presto Pasta with Nori Krinkles

Pasta Power Bowl with Superfoods

❖ ❖ ❖

½ cup spinach and kale, chopped
½ cup mozzarella, shredded
½ cup feta or goat cheese
¼ cup extra-virgin olive oil
2 cups whole-grain pasta, any type
1½ cups tomatoes, chopped
2 teaspoons fresh or dried Italian seasoning
Dash of sea salt and ground pepper
Parmesan, shavings
Pine nuts (optional)

In a mixing bowl, combine spinach, kale, mozzarella, feta or goat cheese, and olive oil. Set aside at room temperature for about 45 minutes. Cook pasta 7–8 minutes. Drain. Place in bowls. Fold in greens and cheese mixture. Mix tomatoes, seasoning, salt, and pepper, put on top of pasta. Sprinkle with Parmesan and nuts.

Makes 3–4 servings.

Linguine with Clam Sauce

❖ ❖ ❖

Clam chowder was a popular dish at a fish restaurant with an ocean view at Newport Beach—a place I lived for a short time. Creamy soups and sauces were something I served as a waitress, but I only fantasized about eating them because I believed they were fattening. (You can rack up calories and sodium, but in moderation, I say, "Soup's on!") And pasta? It did get a bad rap during the high-protein diet food craze. Carbs, past and present, were considered the scourge of dieters. In the film *The Devil Wears Prada*, the character Emily believed carbs were bad, protein was good. Well, these superfood days, the surprise is, you can mix carbs and protein and enjoy the best of both worlds.

⅓ cup Marsala olive fruit oil
1 cup celery, diced
1 carrot, diced
1 onion, chopped
4 garlic cloves (or to taste), chopped
½ cup white wine (optional)
Liquid from canned clams (ignore if you use fresh clams)
Salt, pepper, and cayenne, to taste
½ cup fresh basil and parsley, chopped
12 ounces fresh clams (canned clams may be used if out of season;
    include liquid from canned clams)
1 cup fresh mushrooms, sliced or diced
12 ounces linguine, gemelli, or whole-grain pasta of your choice
Nuts and cheese (your preference) for garnish

In a saucepan, add oil, celery, carrot, onion, and garlic, cook until crisp tender. Add wine, clam liquid, salt, pepper, and cayenne, simmer about 5 minutes. Add basil and parsley, clams, and mushrooms, cook 1–2 minutes. Cook pasta according to package directions, drain, and place in serving platter. Pour sauce and ¼ cup cooking water over pasta, toss gently. Sprinkle with nuts and cheese, if desired.

Makes 4 servings.

(Courtesy: Gemma Sanita Sciabica, from *Cooking with California Olive Oil: Popular Recipes*)

Lobster Mac and Cheese

Back in the sixties, I remember Friday nights. Instead of home-made macaroni and cheese (my mom did make it), she'd dish up the convenient stuff. That means the go-to Kraft mix in the blue box, served with cooked frozen peas or green beans. One night I asked, "Why can't we have the snail-shaped noodles and crunchy bread and tomatoes on top?" She replied, "This weekend I'll fix a nice dinner."

After working all week, to come home for a "second shift" of making a home-cooked meal, well, I get it. She was "whupped," and taking the time to cook up mac and cheese from scratch takes effort. This decadent superfood recipe is for all the moms in the world who want to serve comfort food on a weeknight, but lack the motivation and time to slave over a hot stovetop.

2 cups whole-grain pasta, cooked (Barilla)
1½ cups half-and half
1 cup Parmesan, finely shredded
2 tablespoons European-style butter
Ground pepper and sea salt, to taste
1 cup lobster, cooked, chopped (You can get cooked shellfish from a
    butcher.)
½ cup broccoli, chopped
½ cup panko (Japanese seasoned bread crumbs)
2 Roma tomatoes, chopped
2 tablespoons fresh basil, chopped

In a pan, boil pasta per package directions. Set aside. In a small skillet, heat half-and-half. Add cheese, butter, pepper, and salt. Do not boil. Combine cheese sauce with cooked pasta. Mix well. Fold in cooked lobster and broccoli. Scoop mixture evenly into ramekins. Top with panko. Bake at 350 degrees F for 25 minutes. Sprinkle with tomatoes and basil.

Makes 4 servings.

As simple as this recipe is (except if you choose to cook the lobster yourself; I recommend purchased cooked lobster from your trusty butcher), it is more flavorful and easier on the eyes than the box kind I ate as a kid or even the organic type you can buy in the frozen food aisle at the supermarket. The crunchy garlic-seasoned bread crumbs, scrumptious chunks of shellfish, creamy sauce, and pasta make this super comfort food.

Noodle Salad with Sesame Dressing

❖ ❖ ❖

Exotic salads with sea vegetables, Asian noodles, and nut butter are exciting and fun to eat. This noodle salad is more edgy than macaroni salad because of its superfood ingredients. In the award-winning film *As Good as It Gets*, Jack Nicholson has a line about how not everyone in the world gets to enjoy picnics and eating noodle salad. But with this easy and novel pasta delight, I beg to differ.

FOR THE SALAD

1 cup hiziki or arame (Eden)
¼ cup water
2 medium carrots, julienned
8 ounces (1 package) udon noodles (Asian wheat noodles) (Eden)*
¼ cup green onions, thinly sliced

FOR THE DRESSING

½ teaspoon hot pepper sesame oil (Eden)
1½ teaspoons ume plum vinegar (Eden)
¼ cup organic toasted tahini (sesame butter)
3 cloves garlic, minced

Rinse the hiziki or arame, then soak it in ¼ cup warm water 10–15 minutes. While the sea vegetable is cooking, lightly steam carrots, 1–2 minutes. Rinse with cold water to set color and set aside. Cook noodles as package directs, rinse, and drain. When the arame or hiziki is done, mix with the carrots, noodles, and green onions in a medium bowl. To prepare dressing, blend all ingredients in a blender or food processor, add to salad, and mix well. Serve chilled or at room temperature.

*Noodles can be found from Eden online, in the Asian foods section at a supermarket, or at a specialty Asian shop.

(Courtesy: Eden Foods)

Presto Pasta with Nori Krinkles

❖ ❖ ❖

Once again, I'm dishing up a sea vegetable dish paired with pasta (a different variety of the common superfood) because both are superfoods and may attract the adventurous diner. And since it's prepared in a creative way with familiar superfoods, such as broccoli flavored with scallions, you'll enjoy this easy-to-make dish for yourself, your family, your friends. Soba noodles can be found from Eden online, in the Asian foods section at a supermarket, or at a specialty Asian foods shop.

8 ounces any soba (made with buckwheat flour) or udon noodles
   (Eden)
1 tablespoon shoyu soy sauce, or to taste (Eden)
¼ cup Toasted Nori Krinkles (Eden)
¼ cup carrots, julienned, blanched 1 minute
½ cup small broccoli florets, blanched 2 minutes
¼ cup scallions, chopped fine
1½ teaspoons toasted sesame oil (Eden)

Cook pasta as package directs, rinse and drain. Toss with soy sauce, nori, carrots, and broccoli. Serve garnished with scallions and oil. Serve with a pot of tea and almond butter cookies (see "Super Desserts" for recipe).

(Courtesy: Eden Foods)

Super Entrees

Superfoods used in main dishes, whether they are fish, poultry, or vegetables, are easily found on menus at dives and five-star restaurants. Think fresh, organic, farm-to-table fare (and comfort superfoods, too!) because these are the things attracting millennials and boomers and people in earlier and later generations and generations to follow.

Back in the fifties, in the twentieth century, meat and potatoes were the main meal favorites, including steak and chops paired with French fries or Tater Tots (deep-fried, not baked). But these days, main meals with lean meat and fish can be full of deliciousness. Crispy Fish Fillets in Oatmeal and Lemon Chicken Breasts with Wild Rice and Crucifers can satisfy your appetite and taste buds. The days of red meat and fried vegetables are usually considered to be old school, because fish, poultry, and baked veggies, paired with plenty of fresh herbs and spices, are superfood delights, delicious and good for your health's sake (at any age).

Crispy Fish Filets in Oatmeal
Halibut with Watermelon Sauce
Quinoa Stuff(-ed) Pepper Bowl
Lemon Chicken Breasts with Wild Rice and Crucifers
Stuffed Jumbo Shrimp

Crispy Fish Fillets in Oatmeal

❖ ❖ ❖

Olive oil expert Judy Ridgway shares how this fish recipe plays a role in her life. "In Scotland herring fillets are traditionally fried in a coating of fine oatmeal which gives a wonderful crunchy texture to the fish," she says. Ridgway adds that you should be sure to use extra-virgin olive oil for the frying of the fish to help protect the heat-sensitive omega-3 fatty acids.

1½ pounds mixed fish fillets
Salt and black pepper, freshly ground
Juice of ½ fresh lemon
2 eggs, beaten
4 tablespoons fine oatmeal
Extra-virgin olive oil for frying

Season the strips of fish with plenty of salt and pepper, then sprinkle with the lemon juice. Pour the beaten egg into a bowl and sprinkle the oatmeal onto a plate. Pour the oil into a large frying pan to just cover the base with about ¼ inch of oil. Heat the oil over a medium to high heat. Quickly dip each piece of fish in the egg, then completely coat it with oatmeal. Drop into the hot foil, fry 6–8 minutes, turning once, until the fish is golden brown and crispy. Check the fish to be certain it is completely cooked through, repeat the process with the next batch. Drain the cooked fish onto kitchen paper, keep warm until all the fillets are cooked.

Makes 6–8 servings.

(Courtesy: Judy Ridgway)

Halibut with Watermelon Sauce

It's no secret that millennials like food to be fresh and exotic, whereas baby boomers like to get disease-fighting antioxidants by eating power foods, like the ones in this recipe, from around the year 2000. It offers citrus, egg, fish, nuts, maple syrup, and watermelon—all superfoods (not to forget garlic and olive oil) that can please both generations. It caught my eye, and I sense you'll find it a good catch, too.

2 cups watermelon pieces (or melon of your choice)
2 tablespoons low-sodium soy sauce
¼ cup pure maple syrup or honey
1 tablespoon cornstarch
4 garlic cloves, minced
Salt, pepper, and paprika, to taste
½ cup bread crumbs
¼ cup walnuts, ground
¼ cup parsley, chopped
1 egg white, slightly beaten
¼ cup Marsala olive oil
4 halibut fillets (6 ounces each, about 1-inch thick; can substitute
   any firm white fish.)
2 limes or lemons, in wedges

Blend watermelon, soy sauce, syrup, cornstarch, garlic, salt, pepper, and paprika in a jar or blender. Set aside. In a pie plate, add bread crumbs, walnuts, parsley. In another pie plate, add egg white. Coat fish on both sides in egg white, then in bread crumbs. In a large non-stick skillet, over medium heat, add olive oil. Cook fillets about 4 minutes on each side or until the fish flakes easily when tested with a fork. Remove fillets onto serving platter, cover, keep warm. In a saucepan, bring watermelon mixture to a boil, cook 1 minute, stirring constantly. Pour over halibut, serve with lime wedges.

Makes 4–6 servings.

(Courtesy: Gemma Sanita Sciabica, from *Cooking with California Olive Oil: Popular Recipes*)

Quinoa Stuff(-ed) Pepper Bowl

❖ ❖ ❖

I used to go to Safeway and gaze at the picture on the box of frozen, packaged stuffed bell peppers, an American dish filled with ground beef, white rice, and tomato sauce on top. It took me back to a time when I was a kid and enjoyed my mom's porcupine balls (meatballs with rice sticking out; the stuffed bell peppers were for the grown-ups). Nowadays, going meatless and eating more vegetables and grains is gaining momentum for me—and perhaps, you too. This recipe is inspired by my mom's stuffed peppers, switched up with a twenty-first-century quinoa twist.

1½ cups quinoa, cooked
2 tablespoons European-style butter or olive oil
2 small bell peppers, green and red, chopped
2 tablespoons yellow onion, chopped
1 tablespoon garlic, minced (optional)
Sea salt and ground black pepper, to taste
2 tomatoes, sliced
½ cup mozzarella, grated
4 tablespoons Parmesan, grated
Basil leaves for garnish

In a pan, cook quinoa according to instructions on bag. Meanwhile, in a skillet, melt butter or oil and sauté peppers, onion, garlic, salt, and pepper. Add into quinoa. Place mixture into two baking bowls or ramekins. Top with tomatoes. Sprinkle with mozzarella. Bake at 350 degrees F about 20 minutes. Top with Parmesan. Garnish with basil.

Lemon Chicken Breasts with Wild Rice and Crucifers

I can recall, one summer while living in the Santa Cruz Mountains, making fried chicken and salad with leafy greens. It was the only poultry dish I knew was fail-proof. I quickly browned chicken breasts in a frying pan, then popped the poultry into the oven. While the chicken was baking, I took my two Labrador retrievers down to the river for a quick romp. The chicken was overcooked. Like an embarrassed chef competing on a Food Network challenge segment, I had worked against the clock to impress the judges. This bird dog–inspired recipe is a keeper, but do not let it go to the dogs!

FOR THE CHICKEN

4 chicken breasts, free range, organic
¼ cup whole-wheat flour (King Arthur)
½ cup olive oil
¼ cup fresh basil, chopped
¾ cup fresh lemon juice
Sea salt and pepper, to taste
1 teaspoon Italian spices
Lemon slices and parsley for garnish

FOR THE RICE AND CRUCIFERS

1 cup wild rice (or brown rice)
2 cups organic chicken broth
1 cup broccoli and cauliflower, chopped
2 tablespoons each olive oil and European-style salted butter, melted

Coat chicken breasts with flour. Put poultry in a roasting pan. Drizzle with olive oil. Bake about 20 minutes at 350 degrees F. Turn breasts once. Take chicken out of the oven, top with basil, juice, salt, pepper, and Italian spices, place back into oven for about 25 minutes or until poultry is golden brown.

Cook the rice in chicken broth per directions on package. While rice is simmering, stir-fry vegetables in oil and butter, 3–4 minutes. Place rice on a serving plate, top with chicken breasts and vegetables. Garnish with lemon slices and parsley

Makes 4–6 servings.

Stuffed Jumbo Shrimp
❖ ❖ ❖

Shellfish is a food I link to Fisherman's Wharf in San Francisco and Pike Place Market in Seattle. Shrimp louie is a common dish I adore on the waterfront in any coastal town and enjoy preparing at home in the mountains. Gemma Sanita Sciabica has shellfish recipes, like this one, that are fail-proof. Add artisanal whole-grain bread and leafy green salad, and you've got a big meal to love.

½ cup bread crumbs
Salt, white pepper, and paprika, to taste
¼ cup Romano, grated
4 garlic cloves, minced
1 egg white
⅓ cup fresh basil, parsley, or cilantro, minced
¼ cup pine nuts or currants
1½ pounds jumbo shrimp
¼ cup Marsala olive fruit oil
⅓ cup lime or lemon juice

In pie plate or bowl, combine bread crumbs, salt, pepper, paprika, cheese, garlic, egg white, basil, and pine nuts. Cut cleaned shrimp (leaving tail) along back curve. Open, clean, press flat, and stuff shrimp with bread-cheese mixture, close shrimp with small poultry pins. Arrange shrimp on greased baking dish, drizzle with olive oil and juice. Bake 12–15 minutes at 350 degrees F or until shrimp turn pink. Do not overcook.

(Courtesy: Gemma Sanita Sciabica, from *Cooking with California Olive Oil: Treasured Family Recipes*)

Super Desserts

Sweet desserts can and do include superfoods. In the twentieth century, cakes and cookies were not as healthy because more rather than less sugar was used. Also, lard was common instead of olive oil as a fat, as was frosting out of a box rather than canned fruit.

In the superfoods century, we're dishing up nature's sweets and making super desserts healthier. Almond Butter Crunch Cookies use nut butter, and the EVVO Lemon Cake calls for extra-virgin olive oil and fresh lemon juice. These back-to-nature choices give you dessert, but it's switched up to give you the healing powers of superfoods with a sweet touch.

Almond Butter Crunch Cookies
Apple Crumble
Boysenberry Cobbler
EVVO Lemon Cake

Almond Butter Crunch Cookies

Almonds are plentiful in the Golden State, California. Not only are almonds good for you, they also are a versatile superfood that can be cooked and baked in a wide variety of ways. Some people tell me they don't like to munch on raw almonds because the nut is too hard. Using almond butter, like in this recipe, is a way to get your almonds and eat them, too. These cookies are ideal to pair with any of the smoothies.

FOR THE ALMOND BUTTER

1⅓ cup whole natural almonds
¼ teaspoon salt
4½ tablespoons almond or vegetable oil

FOR THE COOKIES

1 cup almond butter
½ cup butter, softened
1 cup light-brown sugar, packed
1 large egg
½ teaspoon almond extract
1½ cups flour
½ teaspoon baking soda
½ teaspoon salt
½ cup natural California almonds, roasted, chopped

In food processor, for the almond butter, grind almonds, and salt until fine. With motor running, add oil in a slow, steady stream until almond butter forms. Makes 1 cup.

Preheat oven to 350 degrees F. Cream together almond butter, butter, brown sugar, egg, and almond extract until light and fluffy. Combine flour, baking soda, and salt. Blend into creamed mixture. Stir in chopped almonds. Form into 1-inch balls. Place on ungreased cookie sheet and flatten with a fork. Bake 15 minutes, until lightly browned. Cool on wire rack and store in airtight container.

Makes approximately 4 dozen cookies.

(Courtesy: Almond Board of California, *Almonds Are in the Kitchen*)

Apple Crumble

Munching on a crisp, cold fresh apple is a super stress releaser, but savoring a serving of hot apple dessert is comfort food with a capital C. Making an apple pie, if you include a homemade crust, takes time, whereas a fresh fruit crumble is easier and faster to put together and tastes superb, especially if you include plenty of spices to warm up to fall.

FOR THE FRUIT MIXTURE

2 cups Granny Smith apples (4–5 apples), washed, peeled, cored, sliced
½ cup premium orange juice or apple juice
¼ cup maple sugar (Crown Maple)
2 tablespoons European-style butter, melted
1 teaspoon pure vanilla extract
1 teaspoon cinnamon
1 teaspoon allspice
Juice of 1 lemon

FOR THE CRUMBLE TOPPING

½ cup oats
¼ cup maple sugar (Crown Maple)
¼ cup European-style butter
Vanilla bean gelato or vanilla Greek yogurt

Preheat oven to 350 degrees F. Put apples in a bowl. Add juice, sugar, butter, vanilla, cinnamon, allspice, and lemon juice. Set aside in refrigerator. In another bowl, combine oats, sugar, and butter. The mixture should be moist and form crumbled balls. (Add more butter to get the right consistency if needed.) Dish fruit high into two or three ramekins. Top with crumble topping. Place in a pan filled half with water. Bake in oven about 1 hour. (Turn the oven up to 425 degrees F for the last 20 minutes.) Once the crumble is light brown and fruit bubbly, it's done. Serve warm with gelato.

Makes 2–4 servings.

Boysenberry Cobbler

All berries are sweet, juicy, and nutritious. It's blackberries, though, that have won me over for years. Oregon blackberry sherbet, like Henry Fonda ordered in the classic film *Guess Who's Coming to Dinner*, makes me want to join him. Also, my mom used to make a summertime berry cobbler that could take you back to hot nights, kids playing hide-and-seek, and the sound of an ice cream truck driving down the street. It's one of those nostalgic desserts that'll melt your heart every time it's dished up in a bowl with a dollop of creamy, cold homemade vanilla ice cream. You can use frozen blackberries if you can't find boysenberries. It's worth purchasing the pricey ones in the off season, or waiting until summer to enjoy this dessert that pleases the palate at any age.

FOR THE FRUIT

4 cups boysenberries or blackberries, fresh (try Trader Joe's or
    Safeway)
¼ cup sugar
¼ cup flour

FOR THE TOPPING

½ cup flour
¼ cup sugar
¼ cup walnuts
2 tablespoons fresh lemon juice
Vanilla Greek yogurt or vanilla ice cream for garnish
Dark-chocolate shavings for garnish (optional)

In a mixing bowl, combine berries with sugar and flour. Do not over mix. Place into ramekins. Mix flour, sugar, nuts, and lemon juice for the topping. Drop topping over the berries. Bake cobbler approximately 30 minutes or until berries are bubbling and topping is golden brown. Cool. Serve with vanilla Greek yogurt or ice cream. Sprinkle with dark-chocolate shavings.

Makes 4 servings.

EVVO Lemon Cake

❖ ❖ ❖

The folks at the North American Olive Oil Association report that this amazing lemon cake got rave reviews when they shared it with nutritionists and dietitians at their booth at a recent Food & Nutrition Conference & Expo. The chefs at the Westin O'Hare hotel created the cake for the conference, and they allowed the association to share this recipe.

¾ cup extra-virgin olive oil plus additional oil for greasing a pan
1 large lemon
1 cup cake flour (not self-rising)
5 large eggs, separated; reserve 1 white for another use (eggs should
    be room temperature)
¾ cup plus 1½ tablespoons sugar
½ tablespoon salt

Put oven rack in middle position and preheat oven to 350 degrees F. Grease 9-inch pan with oil, then line bottom with a round of parchment paper. Oil the parchment. Finely grate enough lemon zest to measure 1½ teaspoons and whisk together with flour. Halve lemon, then squeeze and reserve 1½ teaspoons fresh lemon juice. Beat together yolks and ½ cup sugar in a large bowl with an electric mixer at high speed until thick and pale, about 3 minutes. Reduce speed to medium and add olive oil (¾ cup) and reserve lemon juice, beating until just combined (mixture may appear separated). Using a wooden spoon, stir in flour-zest mixture (do not beat) until just combined.

Beat egg whites (from 4 eggs) with ½ teaspoon salt in another large bowl with cleaned beaters at medium-high speed until foamy, then add ¼ cup sugar a little at a time while beating, and continue to beat until egg whites just hold soft peaks, about 3 minutes. Gently fold one third of whites into yolk mixture to lighten, then fold in remaining whites gently but thoroughly.

Transfer batter to pan and gently tap pan against work surface once or twice to release any air bubbles. Sprinkle batter evenly with remaining 1½ tablespoons sugar. Bake until puffed and golden and a wooden pick or skewer inserted in center of cake comes out clear, about 45 minutes. Cool cake in pan on a rack, about 10 minutes, then run a thin knife around the edge of the pan and remove the side of the pan. Cool cake to room temperature, about 11/4 hours. Remove bottom of pan and peel off parchment, then transfer cake to a serving plate.

Makes approximately 10 servings.

(Courtesy: North American Olive Oil Association, www.aboutoliveoil.com.)

FINAL SUPERFOODS NOTES

When I embarked on the journey into Superfoodsland, I thought my diet was super, right? Not so much. I discovered that my food choices were lacking in protein, had too many hidden sugars, and that sodium was one of my guilty pleasures. But now, my fridge and pantry have been revamped. There's a balance of superfoods—not just bunny grub. It was a worthwhile adventure, taking me out of my normal diet comfort zone.

These days, kale—not just baby spinach—is in the vegetable bin in my refrigerator. I'm using more whole-grain pasta shapes and sizes and cooking up one-bowl dishes (with fresh spices and herbs for flavor to whisk me off to different cultures) and using a lot of superfruits, nuts, and seeds in smoothies.

The berries in my diet are no longer just strawberries from Watsonville, California; fresh blackberries and dried cranberries (not just during Thanksgiving) are also some of my favorite superfruits in both smoothies *and* salads. Yes, I finally learned to love leafy green salads with vegetables and fruits, even a bit of avocado. And I love having my super blender with a lot of frills, from "puree" to "grate" settings. (I confess I didn't buy an ice cream maker, but I do purchase the all-natural brands of gelato and ice cream and add superfoods.)

During the writing of this seventh book in the *Healing Powers* series, the commercialization of nature's finest superfoods, I have become more aware of the gentrification, deforestation, use of pesticides on our sacred hardworking honeybees that pollinate our superfoods, and pollution in our oceans, all of them rude reminders of what is happening to my world—and yours too. But buying organic foods, eating sustainable superfoods, going green, and liking clean food versus processed eats is becoming a way of life for people (of all ages) in the twenty-first century—and this difference is a super thing, as is going back to nature.

Garden of Apples

During one early October, harvest season time in California, I envisioned going to an out-of-town farm in Placerville (about an hour away from Lake Tahoe) to pick apples off trees. As a birthday present, my younger sibling and I took the trip to Apple Hill. We both had images of meeting a friendly farmer who'd take us on a tractor followed by a couple of herding dogs. The early autumn sunshine would warm us up while we carried baskets to fill with big, fresh apples. We'd climb on stools and pick nature's finest fruit. Excited about the rural experience awaiting us, we drove down the winding road, off the hill, anticipating apple orchards, and the Neil Young song "Harvest Moon" was playing in my head. But there was a little glitch.

We didn't see apples on trees. Not one. A big sign read: "No apple picking." We left and drove up the road, but the farms and small stores all had signs reading "Closed." Locals told us, "Tourists can't pick apples." We ended up at a busy tourist attraction. Pumpkins and Christmas trees were visible and for sale, as was barbecue, ice cream, and pricey fruit—including apples—in an indoor-outdoor store chock-full of families and lots of children.

Disappointed amid tourists and no open apple farms, we drove back up to the hill. I ended up at Safeway and picked up a bag of organic apples at a good price. Later, I discovered I wasn't the only one who had endured such a wild ride at the apple haven. I was told by the apple organization that it had been a busy harvest time and we had come late in the season—and going on a weekday wasn't a wise move, either. There were farms, though, that did offer apple picking, but we had missed the apple boat. So, my fantasy remains in my imagination until next year.

Remember, I grew up in San Jose back more than a half century ago when the population was fifty-one thousand—not the millions now in Silicon Valley. *The Healing Powers of Superfoods* is for you to know which superfoods are healing for you—even if you cannot go outdoors and pick apples or grow a vegetable garden, unless you live on a farm like I told you I did when I was a kid.

Nowadays, it's places like Apple Hill (we could have purchased the ready-picked boxed apples), farmers' markets, health food stores, and supermarkets that all do sell organic produce and superfoods for you to enjoy.

So now you're in the know about which superfoods are super for you—whether you live in the city, suburbs, or a rural region in the United States or around the world. Despite changes to Earth due to man's tampering and nature's wrath, we still can enjoy nature's healthiest foods. But sometimes you have to go the extra mile to get the real deal.

As you enjoy a fresh salad or sip a smoothie with superfoods and plan your next meal full of whole, clean fare, I leave you with some simple words of wisdom from the good doctor of yesteryear. Hippocrates says it best: "If we could give every individual the right amount of nourishment and exercise, not too little and not too much, we would have found the safest way to health." And it's the powers of superfoods that, much like tea, take me to the place I love—wherever I am. I can tell you (no exaggeration) it's my favorite superfoods that are comforting and make me feel at home.

Superfood Resources: Where Can You Buy Superfoods?

*The secret of success in life is to eat what you like
and let the food fight it out inside.*
—MARK TWAIN

As superfoods, especially the classic foods with a twenty-first-century healthful twist, are more popular for mainstream America and around the globe, people like you and me are willing to go the extra mile to find their favorites.

Superfoods such as dried fruits, nuts, seeds, and whole grains are in demand so they can be used and enjoyed year-round. Stored foods can be better than perishables (something to think about during winter months and if you don't want to waste fresh superfoods, which can spoil quickly if not used fast enough).

Here is a superfoods shopping list of my personal favorite go-to places. As times goes on, a variety of classic oldies and "new" upcoming superfoods may be game changers; however, most will still be readily available. You can find your all-natural, organic superfoods at super-centers like Whole Foods Markets and Trader Joe's, farmer's markets, cafes and restaurants, online stores, specialty shops, and health food stores (good for exotic superfoods such as nut butters, protein powders, sea vegetables, and seeds) around the nation and globe.

Don't be disappointed if some big companies merge with others as time passes or if smaller companies may be gone due to different reasons. But if that happens, simply try another similar company and experience the novelty, and you may be pleasantly surprised. Change is part of life, and superfoods are not excluded. If you discover your resource is AWOL or has added or deleted an ingredient in a superfood, think of it as a positive change (more times than not) in the world of Superfoodsland.

SUPERFOOD COMPANIES

Gold Mine Natural Food Company
13200 Danielson Street, Suite A-1
Poway, CA 92064
www.goldminenaturalfoods.com

This company offers plant-based and organic foods. They carry a wide variety of natural, organic superfoods.

Sciabica's California Olive Oil
2150 Yosemite Blvd.
Modesto, CA 95354
www.sunshineinabottle.com

Sciabica specializes in cold-pressed olive oils (another superfood to pair with the superfoods in this book) using varieties of California olives. (I have included recipes throughout the book that have been created by Gemma Sanita Sciabica using their products.)

SPECIALTY FOODS

Eden Foods, Inc.
701 Tecumseh Road
Clinton, MI 49236
www.edenfoods.com

Specialty items include a wide variety, such as ancient grains (muesli to pasta such as Spinach Spirals), apple butter spread, dried fruits (Spicy Berry Mix, Dried Cranberries, Dried Montmorency Cherries, Dried Wild Blueberries, and Wild Berry Mix), nuts (Tamari Roasted Almonds), sea vegetables, and seeds (Roasted and Salted Pumpkin Seeds, Tamari Roasted Spicy Pumpkin Seeds).

King Arthur Flour
Bakery, Café, Store, and School
135 U.S. Rt. 5 South
Norwich, VT 05055
www.kingarthurflour.com/shop

Specialty items for all of your cooking and baking needs, including whole-grain flour.

Lake Champlain Chocolates
750 Pine Street
Burlington, VT, 05402
www.lakechamplainchocolates.com

Offers quality chocolate (up to 80 percent cacao content), including chocolate with real maple syrup, dried fruits, nuts, nut butter, and seeds.

HEALTH ORGANIZATIONS

American Cancer Society
www.cancer.org

Academy of Nutrition and Dietetics
www.eatright.org

American Heart Association
www.heart.org

Superfood Organizations

Almond Board of California
1150 Ninth Street, Suite 1500
Modesto, CA 95354
www.AlmondBoard.com

The American Egg Board
www.aeb.org
North American Olive Oil Association
3301 Route 66, Suite 205, Bldg. C
Neptune, NJ 07753
www.aboutoliveoil.org

This association is committed to supplying North American consumers with quality products in a fair and competitive environment, providing an understanding of the various grades of olive oil, and providing information about the benefits of olive oil in nutrition, health, and the culinary arts.

As of this writing, I find that manufacturers and retail outlets are gaining momentum and joining the super superfoods train, whereas, a book titled *The Healing Powers of Superfoods* is both timely and timeless. More manufacturers could be added to this book, but because of the growing demand and the new superfoods to choose from, it is impossible to include more established and upstart companies marketing such products.

Notes

CHAPTER 1:
THE POWER OF SUPERFOODS

1. Julie Morris, *Superfood Smoothies: 100 Delicious, Energizing & Nutrient-Dense Recipes* (New York, NY: Sterling Publishing, 2013), 16.
2. David Wolfe, *Superfoods: The Food and Medicine of the Future* (Berkeley, CA: North Atlantic Books, 2009), 1.
3. Steven G. Pratt, M.D., and Kathy Matthews, *SuperFoods Rx: Fourteen Foods that Will Change Your Life* (New York, NY: HarperCollins, 2004), 6.

CHAPTER 3:
APPLES

1. Jonny Bowden, Ph.D., C.N.S., *The 150 Healthiest Foods on Earth: The Surprising, Unbiased Truth About What You Should Eat and Why* (Beverly, MA: Fair Winds Press, 2007) 93.
2. A. D. M. Briggs, A. Mizdrak, and P. Scarborough. "A Statin a Day Keeps the Doctor Away," *BMJ* (December 17, 2013): 347, doi:10.1136/bmj.F7267.
3. G. M. Huber and H. P. Rupasinghe, "Phenolic Profiles and Antioxidant Properties of Apple Skin Extracts," *Journal of Food Science* 74 (2009): C693–C700, doi:10:1111/j.1750-3841.2009.01356.x.
4. Christina W. Moyle, et al., "Potent Inhibition of VEGFR-2 Activation by Tight Binding of Green Tea Epigallocatechin Gallate and Apple Procyanidins to VEGF: Relevance to Angiogenesis,"

Molecular Nutrition & Food Research 59, no. 3 (2015); 401–12, doi:10.1002/mnfr.201400478.

5. Editors of FC&A Medical Publishing, *The Folk Remedy Encyclopedia: Olive Oil, Vinegar, Honey and 1001 Other Home Remedies* (Peachtree City, GA: Frank W. Cawood and Associates, Inc., 2004), 155.

Chapter 4:
Berries

1. Kenneth F. Kiple, *The Cambridge World History of Food*, vol. 2 (Cambridge University Press, 2000) 1731–32

2. Liz Applegate, *101 Miracle Foods that Heal Your Heart* (Paramus, N.J.: Prentice Hall Press, 2000), 81.

3. Cal Orey, *The Healing Powers of Chocolate* (New York: Kensington, 2010), 73–74.

Chapter 5:
Cheese

1. http://www.ldfa.org/news-views/media-kits/cheese/history-of-cheese.

2. Applegate, *101 Miracle Foods*, 107.

3. G. Kwon, J. Lee, Y. H. Lim, "Dairy Propionbacterium Extends the Mean Lifespan of *Caenorhabditis elegans* via Activation of the Innate Immune System," *Scientific Reports* (August 17, 2016), doi:10.1038/scirep31713.

Chapter 6:
Crucifers (and Leafy Greens)

1. Vegetables—University of Saskatchwan.agbio.usask.ca. Retrieved 2017-7-11.)

2. Martha Clare Morris, et al., "Nutrients and Bioactives in Green Leafy Vegetables and Cognitive Decline," *Journal of Neuroscience* (December 20, 2017), doi: http://doi:org/10:1212//.

CHAPTER 7:
EGGS

1. Harold McGee, *McGee on Food and Cooking* (London, UK: Hodden and Stoughton, 2004), 70.
2. Don R. Brothell and Patricia Brothell, *Food in Antiquity: A Survey of the Diet of Early Peoples* (Baltimore, MD: Johns Hopkins Press, 1997), 54–55.
3. F. B. Hu, et al., "A Prospective Study of Cardiovascular Disease in Men and Women," *Journal of the American Medical Association* 281 (1999): 1387–94.

CHAPTER 8:
GREEK YOGURT (AND GELATO)

1. Applegate, *101 Miracle Foods*, 294.
2. U.S. Department of Agriculture, National Nutrient Database for Standard Reference (SR21).
3. Lukas Van Oudenhove, et al., "Fatty Acid-Induced Gut-Brain Signaling Attenuates Neural and Behavioral Effects of Sad Emotion in Humans," *Journal of Clinical Investigation* 121, no. 8 (2011), 3094–99. Published online June 25, 2011.

CHAPTER 9:
LEMONS

1. Bowden, *150 Healthiest Foods on Earth*, 124.
2. Ibid., 125.

CHAPTER 10:
MAPLE SYRUP

1. Vimal B. Maisuria, Zeinab Hosseinidoust, and Nathalie Tufernkji. "Polyphenolic Extract from Maple Syrup Potentiates Antibiotic Susceptibility and Reduces Biofilm Formation of Pathogenic Bac-

teria," *Applied and Environmental Microbiology* 81, no 11 (March 27, 2015), doi:10:1128/AEM.00239-15.

2. Sebastien Cardinal, et al., Anti-inflammatory Properties of Quebecol and Its Derivatives," *Bioorganic & Medicinal Chemistry Letters* 25, no. 2 (2016): 440–44.

CHAPTER 11:
NUTS AND NUTTY BUTTERS

1. Almond Board of California, *Almonds in the Kitchen* (Sacramento, CA: Signature Press, 2001), 6.
2. Ibid., 7.
3. Orey, *Healing Powers of Chocolate*, 82–83.
4. Steven G. Pratt, M.D., and Kathy Matthews, *SuperFoods HealthStyle: Simple Changes to Get the Most Out of Life for the Rest of Your Life* (New York: Harper, 2007), 281–82.

CHAPTER 12:
PASTA (WHOLE GRAIN)

1. G. Pounis, et al., "Association of Pasta Consumption Body Mass Index and Waste-to-Hip Ratio: Results from Moli-Sani and INHES Studies," *Nutrition and Diabetes* 6, no. 7 (2016): e218, doi:10.1038/nutd.2016.20.

CHAPTER 13:
PIZZA (WITH TOPPINGS)

1. S. Gallus, et al. "Does Pizza Protect Against Cancer?" *International Journal of Cancer* 107, no. 2 (November 1, 2003): 283–84.

CHAPTER 16:
SEAWEED

1. Orey, Cal. *Doctors' Orders: What 101 Doctors Do to Stay Healthy* (New York: Twin Streams, 2002), 257.
2. Ibid., 307.

CHAPTER 20:
WATER (WATERMELON) AND . . .

1. Orey, *Doctors' Orders*, 135.
2. Anne Hardy, "Water and the Search for Public Health in London in the Eighteenth and Nineteenth Centuries," *Medical History* 28, no. 3 (July 1984): 250–82.
3. Orey, *Doctors' Orders*, 135.
4. R.A. and J. McCaffrey. "Plain Water Consumption in Relation to Energy Intake and Diet Quality Among US Adults, 2005–2012," *Journal of Human Nutrition and Dietetics* 29, no. 5 (March 1, 2016): 624–32: doi:10.1111/jhm.12368.
5. Orey, *Doctors' Orders*, 136.

CHAPTER 21:
. . . OTHER HEALTHY BEVERAGES

1. Calorielab.com, "Aojiru: Japanese Kale Drink Is Full of Vitamins and Indescribably 'Healthy' Tasting," http://calorielab.com/news/2008/03/17/1784/.
2. Orey, Cal, *The Healing Powers of Vinegar: A Complete Guide to Nature's Remarkable Remedy* (New York: Kensington, 2016), 85–88.

Chapter 22:
Whole Grains (Ancient Oats and Quinoa)

1. M. Song, et al., "Association of Animal and Plant Protein Intake with All-Cause and Cause-Specific Mortality," *JAMA Internal Medicine* 176, no. 10 (2016): 1453–63.
2. Shengmin Sang and Yi Fang Chie, "Oats Are a Good Source of Soluble Dietary Fiber Especially B-Glucan, Which Has Outstanding Functional and Nutritional Properties," *Molecular Nutrition & Food Research* 61, no. 7 (July 2017): doi:0.1002/mnf.201600715.

Chapter 23:
Age-Defying Superstuff

1. Orey, *Doctors' Orders*, 299–300.

Chapter 24:
Skinny Superfoods

1. L. Condezo-Hoyos, I. P. Mohanty, and G. D. Noratto, "Assessing Non-digestible Compounds in Apple Cultivars and Their Potential as Modulators of Obese Faecal Microbiota in Vitro," *Food Chemistry* 161 (2014) 208–15, doi:10.1016j.2014.03.122.

Chapter 25:
Home Remedies from Your Kitchen

1. Editors of FC&A Medical Publishing, *Folk Remedy Encyclopedia*, 66.
2. Maisuria, Hosseinidoust, and Tufernkji, "Polyphenolic Extract from Maple Syrup."
3. Martha P. Tarazona-Diez, et al., "Watermelon Juice: Potential Functional Drink for Sore Muscle Relief for Athletes," *Journal of Agriculture and Food Chemistry* 61, no. 31 (2013): 7522–28, doi:10:1021/jf400964r.
4. Editors of FC&A Medical Publishing, *Folk Remedy Encyclopedia*, 281.

Selected Bibliography

Almond Board of California. *Almonds in the Kitchen.* Sacramento, CA: Signature Press, 2001.

American Osteopathic Association. *The Journal of the American Osteopath Association.* Chattanooga, TN: 1917–1918.

Bowden, Jonny, Ph.D., C.N.S. *The 150 Healthiest Foods on Earth: The Surprising, Unbiased Truth About What You Should Eat and Why.* Beverly, MA: Fair Winds Press, 2007.

Crown Maple. *The Crown Maple Guide to Maple Syrup.* Text copyright © 2016 Madava Holdings, LLC.

Morris, Julie. *Superfood Smoothies: 100 Delicious, Energizing & Nutrient-Dense Recipes.* New York: Sterling, 2013.

Pratt, Steven G., M.D., and Kathy Matthews. *SuperFoods HealthStyle: Simple Changes to Get the Most Out of Life for the Rest of Your Life.* New York. Harper, 2007.

———. *SuperFoods Rx: Fourteen Foods that Will Change Your Life.* New York, Harper, 2004.

Sciabica, Gemma Sanita. *Baking Sensational Sweets with California Olive Oil.* Modesto, CA: Gemma Sanita Sciabica, 2005.

———. *Cooking with California Olive Oil: Popular Recipes.* Modesto, CA: Gemma Sanita Sciabica, 2001.

————. *Cooking with California Olive Oil: Recipes from the Heart for the Heart.* Modesto, CA: Gemma Sanita Sciabica, 2009.

————. *Cooking with California Olive Oil: Treasured Family Recipes.* Modesto, CA: Gemma Sanita Sciabica, 1998.

Wolfe, David. *Superfoods: The Food and Medicine of the Future.* Berkeley, CA: North Atlantic Books, 2009.

Connect with Us

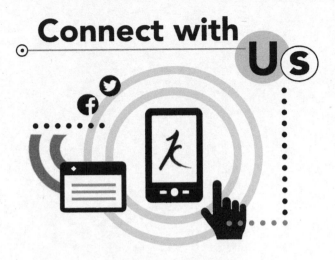

Visit us online at
KensingtonBooks.com
to read more from your favorite authors, see books
by series, view reading group guides, and more.

for sneak peeks, chances to win books and prize packs,
and to share your thoughts with other readers.

facebook.com/kensingtonpublishing
twitter.com/kensingtonbooks

Tell us what you think!

To share your thoughts, submit a review,
or sign up for our eNewsletters, please visit:
KensingtonBooks.com/TellUs.